TALKING TO THE PSYCHIATRIST

ADDICTION

Editing and Proofreading: Randy Saborit Mora

Interior Design, Cover Design and Layout: Otane González Martínez

La Fe Medical Clinic provides medical services and publishes educational and self-help books in the fields of mental health and general medicine, with a human-centered and accessible approach. For more information on how to obtain copies or access additional resources related to emotional health or medical services, please visit our websites:

La Fe Medical Clinic
3030 East 4th Street
Los Angeles, CA 90063
www.lafeclinic.com
www.telegalenos.com
www.miamigodoctor.com

The book Talking to the Psychiatrist: Addiction is part of the Telegalenos a gabacha quitá collection, which has been designed to provide understanding, support and guidance on mental health issues. In simple and warm language, Dr. Alexis Gómez González accompanies the reader through the most common emotional challenges of our time. With the clarity, empathy and clinical experience shown in this collection he seeks to empower the reader to take steps towards their well-being.

Talking to the Psychiatrist: Addiction

Writeen by the Dr. Alexis Gómez González

ISBN: 978-1-968561-14-7

TALKING TO THE PSYCHIATRIST

ADDICTION

ALEXIS GÓMEZ GONZÁLEZ

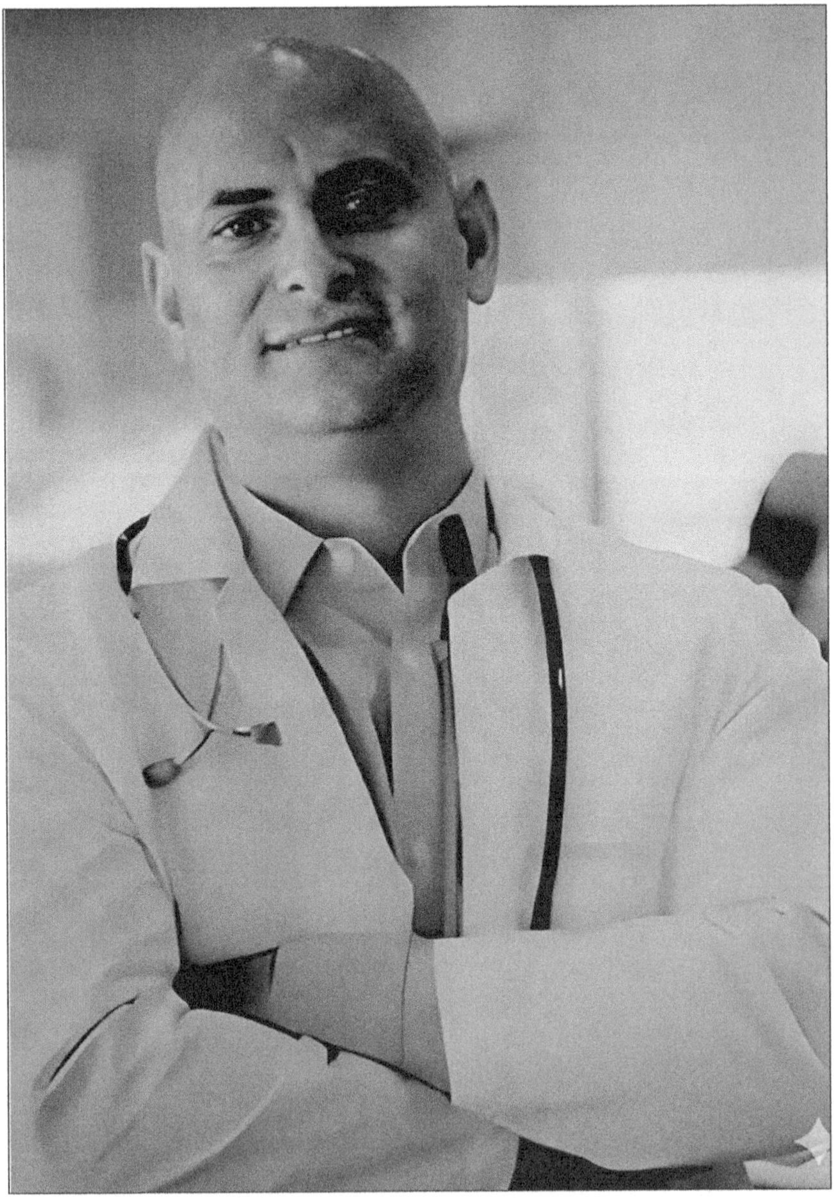

Author's Presentation

My name is Alexis Gómez González. I am a physician who graduated from the School of Medical Sciences of Havana and from the University of Long Beach, California, with a specialty and a master's degree in family medicine and psychiatry. With more than 26 years of clinical, community, and teaching experience in Cuba, Mexico, and the United States, I have worked in the fields of family medicine and psychiatry in diverse communities across these countries, dedicating my career to humanizing medicine and bringing it closer to those who need it most.

I have built my professional life around the comprehensive and compassionate care of individuals with mental health disorders, with particular emphasis on anxiety, depression, insomnia, addictions, and neurodevelopmental disorders. Trained in both medicine and psychiatry, I have combined clinical knowledge with a strong passion for teaching and accessible dissemination. I have created innovative graphic materials and have helped patients, families, and health professionals understand the complexity of the human mind in a clear and empathetic way. I have also worked on developing an approach that integrates science, compassion, and visual language as therapeutic and educational tools.

I currently direct one clinic in Los Angeles and another in Mexico City, both focused on the humanistic and effective treatment of psychiatric conditions, especially in vulnerable populations. I also participate in medical training projects, the creation of illustrated books, and community-based care initiatives.

Acknowledgments

This book would not have been possible without the support and contributions of many people. We are deeply grateful to the mental health professionals, researchers, and experts who shared their knowledge and experience to enrich the content of this work.

Special thanks go to the patients and their families, who allowed their stories to become part of this book, providing an invaluable perspective on the lived experience of addiction.

We also thank our editor and collaborators, whose effort and dedication made the publication of this book possible. Their support was fundamental at every stage of the process.

Finally, we thank all readers who seek to understand and cultivate their emotional intelligence. Your commitment to learning and growth is inspiring and essential to advancing projects and books like this one.

Index

Introduction 21

CHAPTER 1
What is addiction? The Medical, Psychological, and Human Nature of a Misunderstood Disease 23
1.1 Clinical and Social Definition of Addiction 23
1.2 Differences between Use, Abuse, and Dependence 23
1.3 Addiction as a Chronic Brain Disease 24
1.4 Physical Addiction versus Psychological Addiction 24
1.5 Addiction Cycle: from Relief to Deterioration 25

CHAPTER 2
Causes and Origins of Addiction. Childhood, Trauma, Biology, and Culture: the Intertwined Roots of Pain Seeking Relief 27
2.1 Biological, Genetic, and Epigenetic Factors 27
2.1.1 Genetics: a Predisposition, not a Destiny 27
2.1.2 Epigenetics: the Trauma that Marks Genes 27
2.2 Adverse Childhood and Insecure Attachment 28
2.3 Psychological Trauma and Dissociation 29
2.3.1 Chronic Trauma as an Invisible Basis for Addiction 29
2.3.2 Dissociation: internal Exile 29
2.4 Associated Psychiatric Disorders 29
2.4.1 ADHD 29
2.4.2 Depression and Anxiety 30
2.4.3 Bipolar Disorder 30
2.4.4 Personality disorders 30
2.5 Social, Cultural and Family Influences 30
2.5.1 Consumer Cultura 30
2.5.2 Family: Invisible Inheritance 31
2.5.3 Social and Structural Determinants 31
2.6 Final Thought: Addiction Is Not Born, It Is Built 31

CHAPTER 3
What Happens in the Addicted Brain? Neuroscience, Reward Circuits, and Emotional Memory 33
3.1 Dopamine, Glutamate, and the Limbic System: the Desire Triad 33
3.1.1 Limbic System: the Emotional Heart of the Brain 34
3.2 The hijacking of the reward circuit 34
3.2.1 What is the reward circuit? 34
3.2.2 Functional kidnapping 36
3.2.3 From search to conditioning 36
3.3 Tolerance, abstinence, and neuroadaptation 36
3.3.1 Tolerance: the Trick of Repetition 36
3.3.2 Neuroàdaptation: the New Pathological Balance 37
3.4 Brain damage, Neuroinflammation, and Possible Recovery 37
3.4.1 Measurable Brain Damage 37
3.4.2 Chronic Neuroinflammation 37
3.5 Adolescence, Impulsivity and Neurodevelopment 38
3.5.1 The Adolescent Brain: a Construction Site 38
3.6 Final Thoughts 39

CHAPTER 4
Drugs that Trap: Classification and Effects. From the Classic to the Modern: Each Substance and its Trap 41
4.1 Alcohol 41
4.1.1 The Most Dangerous Legal Substance 41
4.1.2 Types of Alcoholic Beverages 41
4.1.3 Alcohol Pharmacology 41
4.1.4 Short-term Effects by Dose 43
4.1.5 Chronic Effects and Multi-organ Damage Brain 43
4.1.6 Fetal Alcohol Spectrum Disorders (FASDs) 44
4.1.7 Diagnosis of Alcohol Dependence Clinical Criteria (DSM-5) 44
4.1.8 Alcohol Use Disorder Identification Test (AUDIT) 44
4.1.9 Examples (selected questions): 45
4.1.10 CAGE Questionnaire 45
4.1.11 Alcohol Withdrawal Syndrome 46
4.1.12 Treatment of Alcoholism 47
4.2 Tobacco and Nicotine 48
4.2.1 The Silent Addiction that Breathes, Hides and Kills 48
4.2.2 Forms of Consumption 48
4.2.3 Nicotine Pharmacodynamics 49
4.2.4 Factors that Increase the Risk of Addiction 49
4.2.5 Immediate Effects 50
4.2.6 Long-term Multisystem Damage 50

4.2.7 Risks in Pregnancy and Childhood 51
4.2.8 Auge of the Vapeo 51
4.2.9 Diagnosis of Nicotine Use Disorder 51
4.2.10 Nicotine Withdrawal Syndrome 53
4.2.11 Omprehensive Treatment 53
4.2.12 Pharmacological Treatment 54
4.2.13 Psychological Support 54
4.3 Marijuana and Cannabinoids 55
4.3.1 Chemical Composition and Cannabis Strains 55
4.3.2 Types of cannabis 57
4.3.3 Forms of Consumption and their Clinical Implications 57
4.3.4 Mechanism of Action: the Endocannabinoid System 57
4.3.5 Acute Effects: between Euphoria and Dysphoria 58
4.3.7 Emotional and Psychiatric Impact 59
4.3.8 Dependence and Abstinence 60
4.3.9 Medical Cannabis: Real Uses and Risks 61
4.3.10 Synthetic Cannabinoids: "The chemist", Spice, K2 61
4.3.11 Cannabis Use Disorder Treatment 61
4.4 Cocaine and Crack Cocaine 62
4.4.1 From Andean Ritual to Urban Collapse 62
4.4.2 Types, Street Names and Forms of Consumption 63
4.4.3 Neurobiology: The Synaptic Storm 63
4.4.4 Sharp Effects (Minute by Minute) 64
4.4.5 Medium and Long-term Medical Consequences 64
4.4.6 Addictive Cycle and Compulsive Behavior 65
4.4.7 The World of Crack: Marginality, Prison and Death 65
4.4.8 Abstinence and Craving 66
4.4.9 Treatment of Cocaine and Crack Use Disorder 67
4.4.10 Maintenance Therapies 67
4.5 Amphetamines and Methamphetamine 68
4.5.1 Types, Street Names, and Presentations 68
4.5.2 Mechanism of Action: Extreme Neurostimulation 70
4.5.3 Immediate Effects of Consumption 71
4.5.4 Long-term Use: Physical and Psychiatric Effects 71
4.5.4.1 Physical Effects 71
4.5.4.2 Psychiatric Effects: 71
4.5.5 Neurocognitive Impact 72
4.5.6 Associated Behaviors 72
4.5.7 Abstinence and Craving 72
4.5.8 Comprehensive Treatment 73
4.5.8.1 Psychiatric Emergencies 73
4.5.8.2 Psychotherapy 73

4.5.9 Pharmacotherapy under Study 73
4.6 Heroin, Fentanyl, and Opioids 75
4.6.1 The Promise of Relief... that Ends with the Breath 75
4.6.2 General Classification of Opioids 75
4.6.2.1 Administration Routes and Consumer Culture 77
4.6.2.2 Mechanism of action: Trick Pain, Trick the Brain 77
4.6.3 Heroin: the Drug that "Embraces" and Abandons 79
4.6.4 Fentanyl: the Molecule of Silence 79
4.7 Benzodiazepines, Anxiolytics and Lethal Combinations 82
4.7.1 The Relief Trap: How Sleep Becomes Dependency 82
4.7.2 Main Benzodiazepines and Anxiolytics 82
4.7.3 Action Mechanism: the Switch of the GABA System 83
4.7.4 Desired Effects and Correct Clinical Use 83
4.7.5 Side Effects and Harms from Chronic Use 84
4.7.6 Lethal Combinations: Fatal Synergies 84
4.7.7 Benzodiazepine Withdrawal: a Brain Storm 86
4.7.8 Treatment of Benzodiazepine Dependence 86
4.7.9 Adjuvant medication 87
4.8 Inhalants: Active, "Mona", Gasoline, Tiner 87
4.8.1 The Silent Poison: Toxic, Street and Childhood Addiction 87
4.8.2 Substances Used and Street Names 89
4.8.3 Mechanism of Action: Central Nervous System Anesthesia 90
4.8.4 Immediate Effects of Consumption 90
4.8.5 Chronic damage: every Inhalation, a Slow Death 90
4.8.6 Social and Demographic Context 91
4.9 Hallucinogens and Psychedelic Drugs 92
4.9.1 Doors of Perception, Abysses of Mind 92
4.9.2 Classification of Hallucinogens and Psychedelics 93
4.9.3 Mechanism of action: opening the doors of consciousness too wide 94
4.9.4 Immediate Effects of Consumption 94
4.9.5 Psychiatric and Physical Risks 94
4.9.6 Contexts of consumption: Spirituality, Celebration, Self-exploration 95
4.9.7 Treatment of Complications 96
4.10 New Designer Drugs and Emerging Substances 96
4.10.1 The Chaos Lab: the Addiction that Still Has no Name 96
4.10.2 General classification of NPS 96
4.10.3 Observed Clinical Effects 97
4.10.4 Consumption Modes 100
4.10.5 Clinical Approach and Medical Challenges 101
4.10.6 Prevention and Surveillance 101
4.11 Combination Drugs and Polydrug Use Syndrome 101
4.11.1 When the Body Becomes a Lethal Laboratory 101

4.11.2 Common Types of Combinations 103
4.11.3 Pathophysiology of Polydrug Use 103
4.11.4 Clinical Manifestations of Polydrug Use 104
4.11.5 The Special Case of the Speedball 104
4.11.6 Combinations in Current Contexts 104
4.11.7 Treatment of Polydrug Use 105

CHAPTER 5
Addictions without Substance. When the Compulsion is Lodged in the Behavior 107

5.1 Gambling Addiction (Compulsive Gambling) 107
5.1.1 When Chance Becomes Prison: the Brain Trapped in the Promise of Winning 107
5.1.2 What is Gambling Addiction? 107
5.1.3 Neurobiology of the Compulsive Gambler 107
5.1.4 Summary Diagnostic Criteria (DSM-5) 108
5.1.5 Profile of the Pathological Gambler 108
5.1.6 What Triggers it? 108
5.1.7 A Disease without Substance, but with the Same Chains 109
5.1.8 Gambling in History and Art 109
5.1.9 Treatment of Gambling Disorder 110
5.1.10 Gambling Addiction Help Resources 111
5.1.11 Support Groups: Gamblers Anonymous (JA) 111
5.1.12 Specialized public and private centers 111
5.1.13 Emotional Hotlines & Free Consultation 112
5.1.14 Digital Resources and Self-care Apps 113
5.1.15 Family Accompaniment and Support Networks 113
5.2 Sex and Pornography Addiction 113
5.2.1 When Desire Becomes a Prision and Pleasure Loses its Face 113
5.2.2 What is Sex and Pornography Addiction? 114
5.2.3 Neurobiology of Sexual Compulsion 114
5.2.4 Signs and Symptoms 114
5.2.5 Common Triggers 114
5.2.6 Clinical Types of People with Sexual Addiction 115
5.2.7 Associated Psychiatric Disorders 115
5.2.8 Emotional and Relational Damage 116
5.2.9 Reflection in Art, Culture and History 116
5.2.10 Help Resources 119
5.3 Addiction to Technology, Social Media, and Video Games 125
5.3.1 When the Mind Slips Non-stop and the Soul Disconnects from the Present 125
5.3.2 What is Technology Addiction? 126

5.3.3 Neurobiology of Digital Addiction 126
5.3.3.1Types of Technology Addiction 126
5.3.4 How is it Diagnosed? 127
5.3.5 Short- and Long-term Consequences 128
5.3.6 Culture, Art and Social Criticism 128
5.3.7 Help Resources 129
5.4 Shopping Addiction and Impulse Control Disorders 133
5.4.1 When the Desire to Buy Becomes an Escape Mechanism 133
5.4.2 Neurobiology of Impulse 134
5.4.3 Risk Factors 134
5.4.4 Treatments 135
5.4.5 Reflections in Culture and Art 135
5.4.6 Help Resources 137
5.5 Workaholism 138
5.5.1 When Productivity Becomes a Prison 138
5.5.2 Clinical Features 139
5.5.3 Neuropsychological Basis 139
5.5.4 Causes and Risk Factors 139
5.5.5 Treatment and Recovery 140
5.6 Reflections in Culture and Art 140
5.6.1 Help Resources 143
5.7 Food Addiction and Compulsive Eating 144
5.7.1 When Comfort Becomes Prison 144
5.7.2 Definition and Diagnosis 144
5.7.3 Neurobiology Involved 145
5.7.4 Root Causes 145
5.7.5 Physical and Psychological Consequences 145
5.7.6 Comprehensive Treatment 145
5.7.7 Reflections in Culture and Art 146
5.7.8 Help Resources 147

CHAPTER 6
Comprehensive Addiction Treatment. Between Science, Psychotherapy and Human Containment 149
6.1 Diagnostic Assessment and Motivation for Change 149
6.1.1 Dimensions of the Comprehensive Assessment 149
6.1.2 Stages of Motivation to Change (Prochaska and DiClemente Model) 150
6.1.3 Motivational Interviewing: the Art of Respectful Dialogue 151
6.2 Treatment Phases: Detoxification, Rehabilitation and Reintegration 152
6.2.1 First phase: Detoxification (Detoxification) 153
6.2.2 Second Phase: Rehabilitation 153

6.2.3 Phase Three: Reintegration 154
6.2.4 Symbolic Image of the Chapter 155
6.3 Pharmacological Treatments. Which Medications and When? 155
6.3.1 Why Pharmacotherapy in Addictions? 156
6.3.2 General Principles of the Pharmacological Approach 156
6.3.3 Treatment According to Type of Substance 157
6.3.4 Behavioral Addictions (Gambling, Sex, Shopping, Food, Technology) 159
6.3.5 Ethical and Practical Considerations 160
6.4 Effective Psychological Therapies 160
6.4.1 Beyond Abstinence 160
6.4.2 Cognitive Behavioral Therapy (CBT) 161
6.4.3 Eye Movement Desensitization and Reprocessing (EMDR) 163
6.4.4 Mindfulness and Compassion 164
6.5 The Role of Mutual Aid Groups (NA, AA, AL-ANON) 166
6.5.1 Listening to Heal: the Power of Peer Sharing 166
6.5.2 What Are Mutual Aid Groups? 166
6.5.3 Structure and Key Principles 166
6.5.4 The Power of the Shared Word 167
6.5.5 Clinical and Emotional Benefits 167
6.6 Therapeutic Community Models and Residential Centers 168
6.7 Relapse. Prevention, Coping and Resignification 172
6.7.1 Neurobiology of Relapse 172
6.7.3 Relapse Prevention: Tools and Strategies 174
6.7.4 Coping and Resignification after a Relapse 174

CHAPTER 7
Accompanying a Loved One with Addiction. Family, Partner, Children 177
7.1 When Love Turns into Pain 177
7.2 The Relational Wound: Loving Someone Who Self-Destructs 177
7.3 Love that Controls, Love that Annuls Itself 178
7.4 When Love Transforms: Saving Limits 178
7.5 Symbolism: the Red Thread and the Scissors 179
7.6 Resources for Family Members 179
7.6.1 Mutual Aid Groups 179
7.6.2 Recommended Books 179
7.6.3 Specific Therapies 179
7.7 Codependency and Healthy Boundaries 181
7.7.1 What Is Codependency? 181
7.7.2 Neurobiology and Psychodynamics of Codependency 181
7.7.3 Clinical Signs of a Codependent Relationship 181

7.7.4 Family and Transgenerational Origins 182
7.7.5 The Emotional Toll of Codependency 182
7.8 Help versus Enable 182
7.9 Healthy Limits: How, When, and Why? 183
7.10 Strong and Empathetic Communication 183
7.11 Healing Paths for the Codependent Family Member 185
7.12 The Role of the Caregiver, Therapist and Support Network 185
7.12.1 The Caregiver: between Love, Exhaustion and Hope 185
7.12.2 The Therapist: Professional Guide and Compassionate Mirror 186
7.12.3 The Support Network: Invisible but Vital Support 187
7.13 Children and Adolescents with Addicted Parents 188
7.13.1 When Home Becomes Unpredictable 188
7.13.2 Neurobiology of Childhood Trauma 188
7.13.3 Family Dynamics and Types of Child Response 188
7.13.4 Short and Long-term Sequelae 190
7.13.5 Therapeutic and Community Approach 191
7.13.6 Keys to Resilience 192
7.14 Community, Legal, and Emergency Resources 193
7.14.1 When Everything Overflows 193
7.14.2 Immediate Emergency Resources 193

CHAPTER 8
Ethical, Legal and Social Aspects 197
8.1 Criminalization versus Treatment 197
8.2 A Brief History of the Criminalization of Consumption 197
8.3 Sick or Delinquents? The Two Models 197
8.4 International Comparisons 198
8.5 Consequences of Criminalization 198
8.6 Ethics, Humanity, and Reform 199
8.7 Real alternatives: Treatment Instead of Prison 199
8.8 The New Paradigm: Health as Justice 199

CHAPTER 9
Addiction in the Homeless Population. When Marginality, Trauma, and Addiction are Intertwined 201
9.1 A Silenced Reality: Statistics and Forgotten Faces 201
9.2 The Street-Addiction-Street Cycle: a Spiral of Exclusion 201
9.3 Low-cost, High-harm Drugs 202
9.4 Barriers to Access to Treatment 202
9.5 Effective Interventions: between Dignity, Health, and Reality 203
9.6 Ethical Implications and Recommendations 203

CHAPTER 10
Human Rights, Discrimination and Access to Health. Addiction as a Matter of Justice, Dignity and Equity 207
10.1 Stigma as a Form of Structural Violence 207
10.2 Discrimination in Health Systems 207
10.3 Criminalization, Poverty and Exclusion 208
10.4 Human Rights Approach to Mental Health and Addiction 208
10.5 Landmark Cases and International Jurisprudence 208
10.6 Practical Recommendations for an Inclusive Approach 209

CHAPTER 11
School and Community Prevention 211
11.1 Scientific Foundations of Prevention 211
11.2 School Prevention: Beyond "Do not Consume" 212
11.3 Community Prevention: Networks that Protect 213
11.4 The Role of Media and Technology 213
11.4.1 Obstacles and Challenges 213
11.4.2 Proposals for Action 214

CHAPTER 12
Drugs and Culture: Cinema, Art, Literature and Spirituality. Between Fascination, Tragedy and Transcendental Search 217
12.1 Cinema: between Glamour, Criticism and Descent 217
12.2 Literature: Cursed Poets and Intoxicated Novels 218
12.3 Art: Distorted Forms and Transcendental Visions 219
12.4 Music: Euphoria, Loss, and Ritual 220
12.5 Spirituality and Ritual Use of Substances 221
12.6 Final Thought: between Symbol and Risk 222
12.7 Resources to Explore and Understand 222

CHAPTER 13
Medical Aikido Applied to Addiction 223
13.1 What Is Medical Aikido? 223
13.2 Who Is this Approach for? 223
13.3 Medical Aikido Formula for Addiction 2A + 2B + 2C + 2D 224
13.4 Medical Aikido for Family Members and Professionals 226
13.5 The Symbolism of Addiction 226
13.6 Addiction as a Path to Self-knowledge 226

CHAPTER 14
A Proposal for Integrative, Symbolic and Resilient Medicine 229
14.1 What do We Mean by "Integrative Medicine"? 229

14.2 The Role of the Symbolic 230
14.3 Resilience as a Central Axis 230
14.4 Proposal for an Integrative Intervention Model 230
14.5 Possible Challenges and how to Deal with Them 231
14.6 Inspiring Cases 232

CHAPTER 15
Resources in Mexico, the United States and Spain 235
15.1 Resources in Mexico 235
15.2 Resources in the United States 236
15.3 Resources in Spain 236

CHAPTER 16
Treatment Plans, Clinical Examples, and Integrated Therapeutic Guidelines 239
16.1 Treating Addiction as a Complex Neurobiological Condition 239
16.2 What Do We Mean by Comprehensive Treatment? 239
16.3 Neurochemical Profiling-Based Pharmacotherapy (DNP-21 Model) 241
16.4 Clinical Cases 242
16.5 Clinical Guidelines by Substance (Summary) 243

CHAPTER 17
Letters to the Family, Addict, and Therapist 245
17.1 The Therapeutic Value of Letters 245
17.2 Scientific Basis: Why Does It Work? 245
17.3 Suggested Letters: Structure and Narrative Examples 246
17.4 Didactic Workshop: How to Use Cards in Therapy 248

CHAPTER 18
Books, Documentaries, and Resources that can Help You 251
18.1 Why Keep Learning? 251
18.2 Recommended Books 251
18.3 Documentaries and Films to Reflect on 252
18.4 Online Resources 253
18.5 How Do You Know if a Resource Is Good? 253
18.6 What Do I Do with This Info Now? 254

CHAPTER 19
The DNP-21 Model Applied to Addiction 257
19.1 What Is the DNP-21 Model? 257
19.2 Instrument AD-DNP-21-Addiction 258
19.3 Clinical Cases 260
19.4 AD-DNP-21-Neurochemical Profile Questionnaire in Addiction 260

APPENDICES 263

Appendix 1 263

100 Frequently Asked Questions in My Consultation 263

Illustrated Glossary of Terms on Addiction 281

***Telegalenos a gabacha quitá* Collection** 285

Introduction

This book is aimed at psychiatrists, doctors, psychologists, nurses, addicted patients and family members. It seeks to be a comprehensive text on the subject of addiction, with a clinical, human and cultural approach. In its pages you will find detailed explanations about the types of drugs, their physiological effects, the short- and long-term consequences, the specific treatments by substance, the abstinence protocols, historical examples, artistic references, and the tools to transform suffering into resilience.

Importance of Understanding Addiction

Addiction is one of the most misunderstood, punished, and stigmatized diseases in the modern world. It is not a lack of character, nor moral weakness. It is a medical, psychological, and spiritual condition that often develops in early grief and is perpetuated in the search for relief.

Understanding addiction from a scientific and compassionate perspective is the first step to addressing it effectively. This book is an invitation to stop judging and start accompanying.

We live in a paradoxical time: never before have we had so much access to information, technology, medicines, therapies, support networks... And yet, never before have we been so lonely, so anxious, so addicted.

Addiction, today more than ever, is not simply a matter of drugs. It is a question of meaning. Speed addiction. To digital validation. Consumption. To the denial of pain. Anything that prevents us from feeling emptiness or facing the wound.

Writing about addiction today is not a technical act. It is a human, ethical, urgent act. Because behind every addict there is an untold story. A fractured childhood. A battle with the mind. A cry that no one heard.

This book is born not only from knowledge, but from contact with that wounded humanity. With the intention of building bridges between science and the soul, between the clinic and compassion, between neurobiology and the embrace.

If you're a healthcare professional, you'll find tools and language here to better understand the complexity of addiction. Whether you're a patient, a family member, or a loved one, you'll encounter words that maybe no one ever said to you. And if you yourself are struggling, this work is also for you: not like a sentence, but like a map. Not as an absolute answer, but as a compass in the midst of chaos.

I've seen people quit heroin, but not be able to leave their violent partner. I have seen young people who left the glass, but could not bear the silence. I've seen mothers who stopped using, but couldn't forgive themselves. And I have also seen patients hit rock bottom and be reborn. I have seen it with my own eyes.

As a psychiatrist I have not treated diseases: I have accompanied processes. I have learned that there is no addiction without history. That there is no cure without listening. And that behind the drug there is a logic, even if it is painful.

Many patients do not need sermons. They need to be looked at without judgment. They need help to put words to what they have not been able to name. This treatise is born of hundreds of conversations, tears, relapses and rebirths. It is not just theory. It is written with the skin.

CHAPTER 1
What is addiction? The Medical, Psychological, and Human Nature of a Misunderstood Disease

1.1 Clinical and Social Definition of Addiction

Addiction is a **chronic, progressive and recurrent** disease of the brain, characterized by the loss of control over a behavior (consumption of a substance or performance of an activity), accompanied by an intense desire (craving), denial of damage and a progressive dissolution of personal autonomy.

From a medical point of view, the American Psychiatric Association (APA) and the World Health Organization (WHO) define it as a **disorder of the reward, motivation, memory and control system**, which causes a compulsive use of a substance or behavior despite its negative consequences.

From a social point of view, it is a highly stigmatized condition, often misinterpreted as moral weakness, lack of willpower or simple "vice", which prevents many affected from seeking help.

Clinical example

A 48-year-old woman who drinks wine every night and hides the bottles from her family. He has liver problems, but insists that "he only does it to relax".

1.2 Differences between Use, Abuse, and Dependence

Concept	Definition	Clinical example
Application	Occasional, controlled consumption, without negative impact	Person smoking a cigar at sporadic parties

Concept	Definition	Clinical example
Abuse	Repeated use with negative consequences, but still with some control	Teenager who uses marijuana every weekend and lowers his school performance
Dependence (addiction)	Loss of control, compulsion, tolerance, withdrawal, and progressive impairment	Patient who needs daily heroin to function, has crises when trying to quit

The progression is not always linear, but many times **prolonged abuse leads to dependence**, especially if genetic, emotional, or contextual factors are involved.

1.3 Addiction as a Chronic Brain Disease

Neuroimaging studies have shown that addiction produces **structural and functional changes in the brain**, especially in three key areas:

- **Prefrontal cortex:** affects judgment, decision-making, self-control.
- **Nucleus accumbens and limbic system:** overstimulation of the reward system → compulsive search for pleasure or relief.
- **Amygdala and stress axis:** hypersensitivity to emotional distress → use as an escape.

These alterations **are not reversible immediately** after stopping the substance, which explains why **relapse is part of the expected course of the disease**.

Medical analogy:

Just as a diabetic patient needs to control their sugar throughout their lives, a person with addiction must learn to manage their triggers and their relationship with desire.

1.4 Physical Addiction versus Psychological Addiction

Appearance	Physical Addiction	Psychological Addiction
Biobasis	Organic dependence on the substance	Emotional attachment to the effect or ritual
Withdrawal symptoms	Tachycardia, tremors, sweating, seizures	Anxiety, irritability, emptiness, insomnia

Appearance	Physical Addiction	Psychological Addiction
Duration of the syndrome	Days to weeks	Weeks to months or years
Example	Alcohol withdrawal → *delirium tremens*	Compulsive use of pornography to calm sadness

Note: In clinical practice, both forms are intertwined and must be addressed simultaneously.

1.5 Addiction Cycle: from Relief to Deterioration

Addiction does not begin with the search for pleasure, but with the search for relief. In many people, especially with a history of trauma, abandonment, depression or anxiety, consumption appears as a way to calm a pre-existing discomfort. The stages of the cycle are as follows:

1- Emotional or situational trigger: sadness, stress, emptiness.

2- Initial consumption: "I relax", "I disconnect".

3- Positive reinforcement (pleasure) → release of dopamine.

4- Chemical rebound → anxiety, guilt, discomfort.

5- Repeated consumption to avoid discomfort (negative reinforcement).

6- Tolerance: no longer has the same effect.

7- Total dependence: it is needed to live (Figure 1).

Clinical Testimony

"I didn't start drinking for fun. I started to stop crying".

Addiction is **a complex disease that compromises a person's biology**, **mind**, and **environment**. Understanding it requires **breaking with social prejudices** and treating it with the same respect as any other chronic disease. This chapter seeks t**o replace judgment with knowledge, and condemnation with compassion and knowledge**.

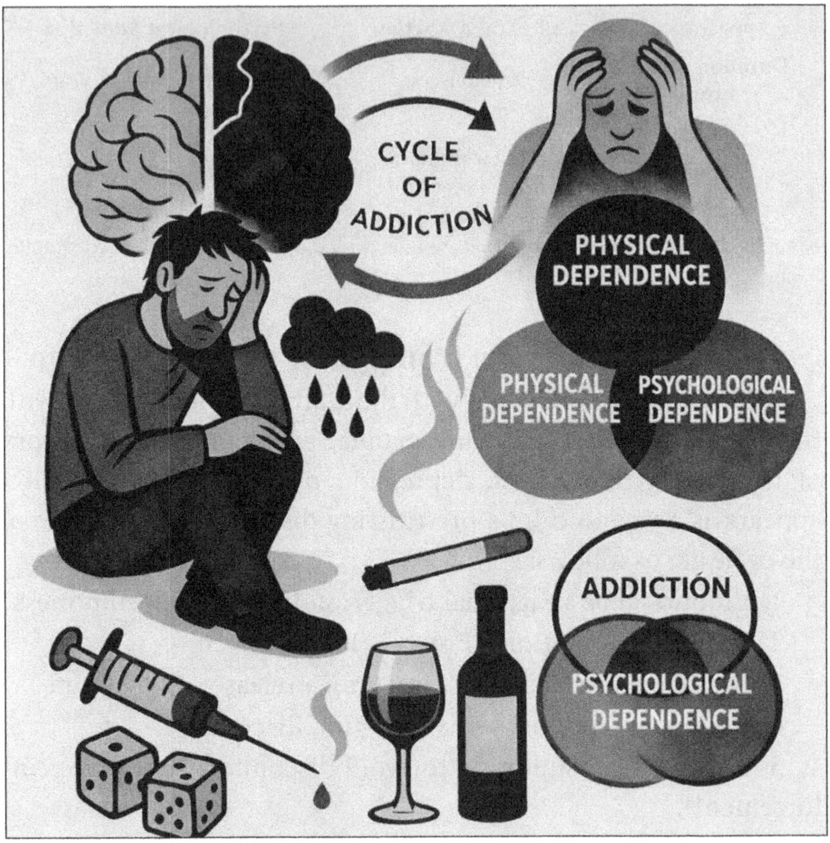

Figure 1. Representation of the addiction cycle. The image shows the interplay between physical addiction and psychological addiction as intertwined dimensions of human suffering. The brain, emotions, substances, and compulsive behaviors form a cycle that traps the individual and highlights both visible and invisible pain. A clear and didactic visual synthesis of the key components of the dependency.

CHAPTER 2
Causes and Origins of Addiction. Childhood, Trauma, Biology, and Culture: the Intertwined Roots of Pain Seeking Relief

2.1 Biological, Genetic, and Epigenetic Factors

2.1.1 Genetics: a Predisposition, not a Destiny

Studies in behavioral genetics reveal that **vulnerability to addiction is partly hereditary**. The current estimate suggests a heritability of **40 to 60%**, influenced by multiple genes affecting:

- **Sensitivity to Dopaminergic Reinforcement**
(e.g., DRD2 gene variants → reduced D2 receptors → lower natural "satisfaction").

- **Impulsivity and executive control**
(genes related to the serotonergic and prefrontal system).

- **Circadian rhythms and emotional regulation**
(relevant in alcoholism and ADHD).

Example: people with the A1 variant of the DRD2 gene tend to experience less pleasure with natural stimuli and a greater response to alcohol or cocaine.

2.1.2 Epigenetics: the Trauma that Marks Genes

Epigenetics explains how the environment "turns on or off" the expression of certain genes without modifying their structure. Childhood trauma, neglect, or chronic stress can:

- Hypermethylate genes related to stress resilience.
- Decrease the expression of GABAergic receptors.
- Permanently alter the **response of the HPA (hypothalamic-pituitary-adrenal) axis.**

This produces **hyperreactive brains**, with greater basal anxiety, hypervigilance and a tendency to **seek out external regulators** such as drugs or compulsive behaviors.

2.2 Adverse Childhood and Insecure Attachment

Adverse Childhood Experiences (ACEs) include:

- Physical, emotional, or sexual abuse.
- Parental neglect.
- Addictions or mental illness at home.
- Separation or imprisonment of a parent.
- Domestic violence or extreme poverty.

People with ≥ 4 ACEs have a 10 times higher risk of alcoholism and 12 times more risk of suicide attempts. A secure attachment is a natural emotional antidote to impulsivity, anxiety, and emptiness. When the child cannot rely on stable care, he or she develops coping strategies that predispose to addiction:

Type of Attachment	Emotional Characteristics	Relationship with Addiction
Anxious	Hypersensitivity to rejection	Obsessive search for approval → use as validation
Avoidant	Emotional suppression, self-isolation	Use of substances to "not feel" or escape contact
Disorganized	Emotional chaos, fear and desire mixed	Impulsive, self-destructive, fragmented behavior

Clinical case

A 33-year-old patient with methamphetamine addiction and compulsive sexual behaviors. History of maternal abandonment, disorganized attachment, and multiple foster homes.

2.3 Psychological Trauma and Dissociation

2.3.1 Chronic Trauma as an Invisible Basis for Addiction

Not all trauma leaves visible scars. Repeated exposure to emotionally crushing experiences generates:

- Fragmentation of the self.
- Disconnection from the body.
- Difficulties in the narrative integration of life.

This predisposes to:

- Use of substances such as "psychic anesthesia".
- Behavioral addictions (pornography, food, gambling) as an escape.
- Dissociative disorders and borderline symptoms with compulsive use.

2.3.2 Dissociation: internal Exile

Dissociation is a protective mechanism against the unbearable. It is expressed as:

- Depersonalization ("it's not me").
- Derealization ("this is not real").
- Loss of time or gaps in consciousness.

The addict often does not seek pleasure, but "to stop being".

Clinical case

Andrea, 28 years old, with a history of intra-family sexual abuse. Benzodiazepine use from the age of 15. "I don't take them to sleep, I take them to disappear".

2.4 Associated Psychiatric Disorders

2.4.1 ADHD

- Dysfunction in the frontostriatal circuit: difficulty in postponing gratification.
- High impulsivity, low tolerance to frustration.

- Early onset of consumption → more severe evolution.

It is estimated that 1 in 3 people with ADHD will develop an addiction if it is not treated properly.

2.4.2 Depression and Anxiety

- Use as self-medication: alcohol or cannabis to "calm down", stimulants to "get out of the hole".
- Substance withdrawal can **worsen the original symptoms**, creating a vicious cycle.

Benzodiazepines are the second most commonly used drug by people with untreated generalized anxiety.

2.4.3 Bipolar Disorder

- Manic phases favor disinhibition, impulsive consumption, spending and risky sex.
- Depressive phases lead to sedation using alcohol, heroin or tranquilizers.
- Incomplete treatment → cyclical pattern of relapses.

2.4.4 Personality disorders

- Especially borderline disorder (BPD): substance abuse as an extension of the identity void.
- Dual behaviors: idealization and destruction, including towards the substance.
- Difficulty in establishing a stable motivation for treatment.

Clinical Testimony

"Drugs don't betray me. Humans do" (patient with BPD and use of glass).

2.5 Social, Cultural and Family Influences

2.5.1 Consumer Cultura

- Alcohol as a ritual in almost all social contexts.

- Tolerance to the use of marijuana as a form of relaxation or creativity.

- Glorification of drugs in music, fashion, cinema, social networks.

"Perico, perico... we turn it on and go to the disco".

2.5.2 Family: Invisible Inheritance

- Consumer parental models: what the child sees, repeats.
- Environments of chaos, violence or denial of the problem.
- Dynamics of codependency, family secrets and taboos.

2.5.3 Social and Structural Determinants

Factor	Impact on Addiction
Chronic poverty	Stress, hopelessness, lack of opportunities
Racism and exclusion	Internalization of inferiority, cultural trauma
Forced migration	Loss of bonds, unprocessed grief
Urban violence	Hypervigilance, early access to drugs
Lack of access to health	Delayed or no diagnosis

2.6 Final Thought: Addiction Is Not Born, It Is Built

No one chooses to have an addiction, but **all systems** (genetic, psychological, social, and cultural) can **conspire to make it happen**. There is no such thing as a "genetic addict" or an "irredeemably traumatized". There are brains in vulnerability and contexts that feed pain.

Treating addiction requires not only **removing the substance**, but also **reconstructing what was not built in childhood, healing what was fractured by trauma**, and **protecting what was made invisible in the culture** (Figure 2).

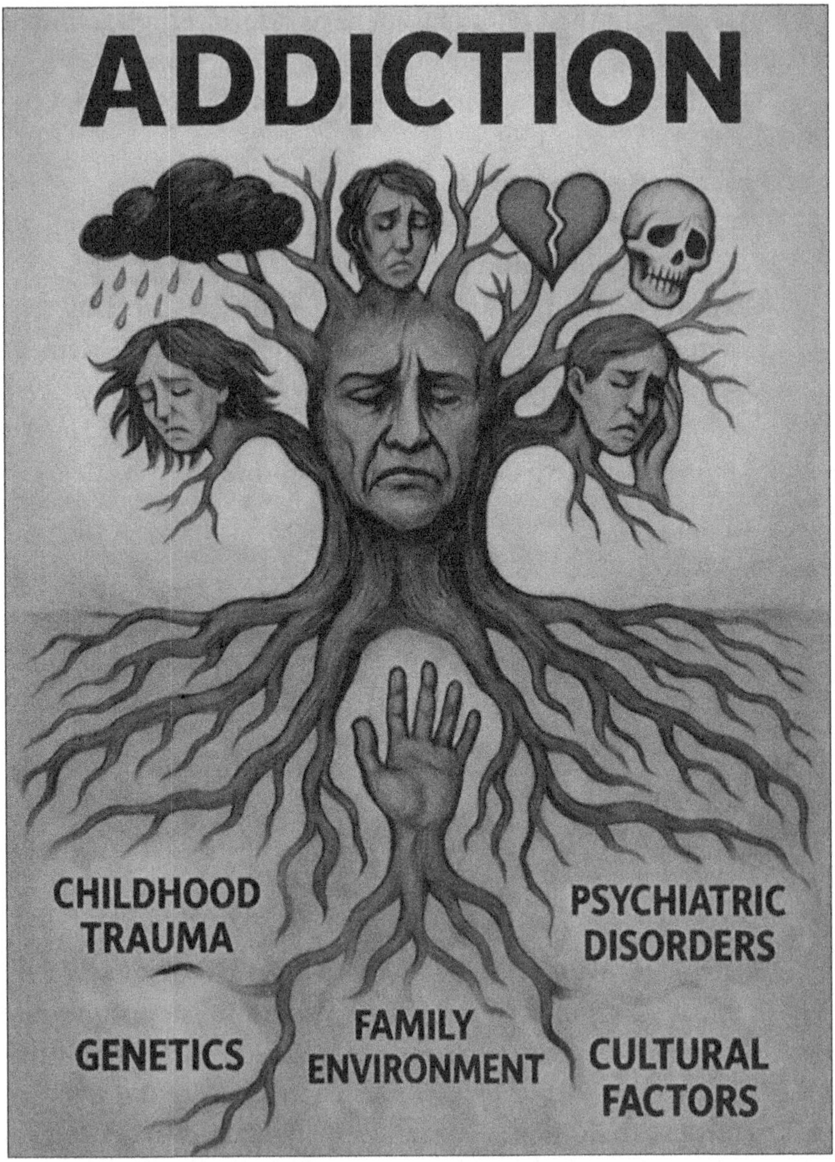

Figure 2. The invisible roots of addiction. This image symbolizes that addiction is not an isolated decision or a moral failing, but the result of multiple deep roots: childhood traumas, dysfunctional family environment, genetic vulnerability, psychiatric disorders, and cultural pressures. The tree, which represents the human being, holds suffering in its trunk and hidden causes in its roots. Healing addiction involves addressing not only the symptom, but also what gave rise to the pain.

CHAPTER 3
What Happens in the Addicted Brain? Neuroscience, Reward Circuits, and Emotional Memory

3.1 Dopamine, Glutamate, and the Limbic System: the Desire Triad

1- Dopamine: the Currency of Motivated Learning

Dopamine is a key neurotransmitter in the reward system, which serves three fundamental functions:

- Positive reinforcement: marks pleasurable experiences (food, sex, achievements).
- Reward memory: Teaches the brain what to repeat.
- Prediction and motivation: it is released even in the anticipation of pleasure.

Under normal conditions, dopamine rises with:

- A sincere hug,
- overcoming a challenge,
- the ingestion of something tasty.

In the addict, those events no longer trigger enough dopamine. **Only the addictive substance or behavior does it**.

Example:

A woman with a cocaine addiction describes how just seeing a white card (similar to the one used to cut coca) makes her heart race. Your brain associates that stimulus with dopamine.

1- Glutamate: the Brain Recorder

Glutamate is the brain's main excitatory neurotransmitter. Along with dopamine, it facilitates:

- learning by conditioning,

- the reinforcement of synaptic connections (LTP–long-term potentiation),
- the association between emotions and contexts.

In addiction, glutamate **strengthens the craving pathways**:

- links a street with consumption,
- a smell with desire,
- an emotion (sadness, anger) with the impulse to use.

This learning is so strong that it persists even after months of abstinence (Figure 3).

3.1.1 Limbic System: the Emotional Heart of the Brain

Key regions:

Region	Function
Nucleus accumbens	Pleasure, anticipatory motivation, euphoria
Amygdala	Emotional association, fear, aversion
Hippocampus	Contextual memory: where, with whom, how
Prefrontal cortex	Judgment, planning, slowing down momentum

The limbic system is the "engine" of desire, but the prefrontal cortex is the "brake". In addiction:

- **The motor is overactive** (high limbic reactivity).
- **The brake is damaged** (weak executive function).

3.2 The hijacking of the reward circuit

3.2.1 What is the reward circuit?

The **mesolimbic dopaminergic system** is a set of brain structures evolutionarily designed to:

- Encourage the search for healthy pleasure.

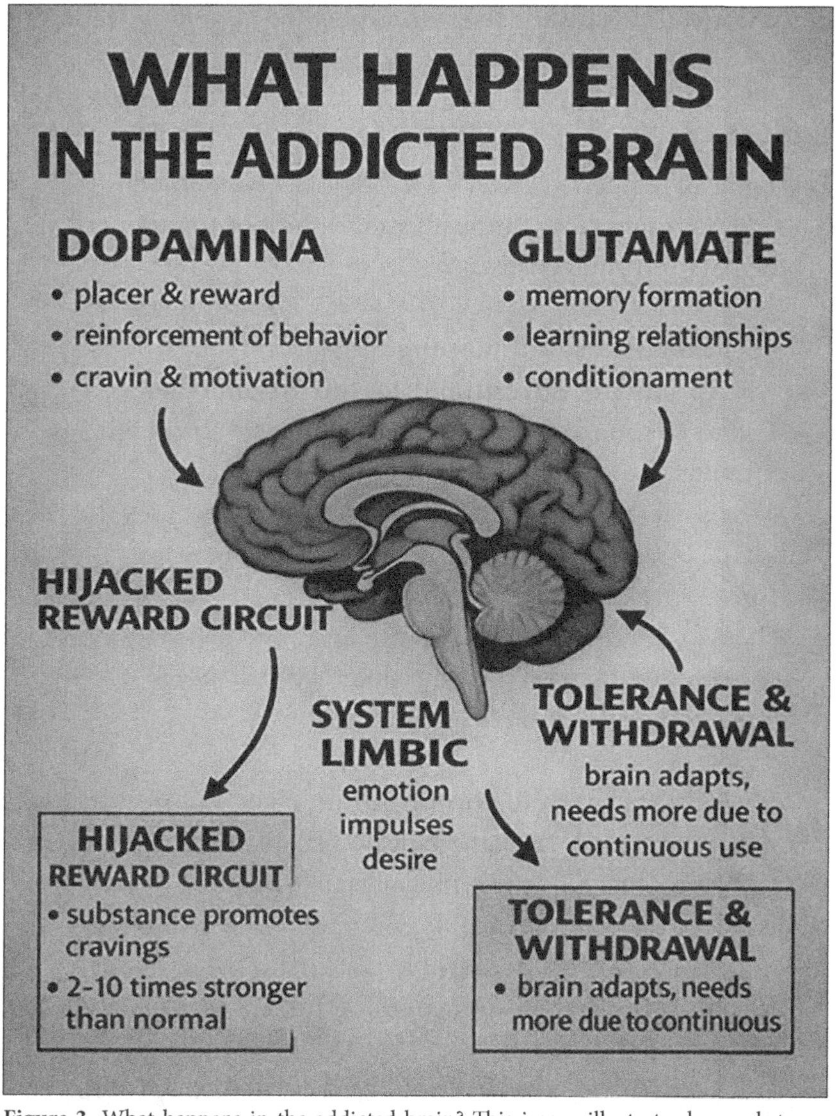

Figure 3. What happens in the addicted brain? This image illustrates how substance use alters the brain's main neurochemical systems: dopamine, which is associated with pleasure, motivation, and reward, and glutamate, which is key to learning and memory. The limbic system, which regulates emotions and impulses, gets caught in a hijacked reward circuit. As consumption progresses, the brain develops tolerance and suffers withdrawal, becoming dependent on the stimulus to function normally.

- Motivate necessary behaviors (feeding, bonding, reproducing).
- Learning by reinforcement.

The key route:

- Ventral tegmental area (VTA) → Nucleus accumbens.
- VTA also projects to the amygdala, hippocampus, and ventromedial prefrontal cortex.

3.2.2 Functional kidnapping

When a substance overstimulates this system:

- Up to 10 times more dopamine is released than with a natural stimulus.
- The system is recalibrated: the substance becomes the "new standard" of pleasure.

Three key consequences appear:

- Loss of interest in other pleasures.
- Motivation focused on obtaining the substance.
- Deactivation of inhibitory judgment.

3.2.3 From search to conditioning

With repeated use, a "pathological" form of learning is activated:

- Craving does not need the substance present: an associated signal (cigarette, voice, place) is enough.
- The system enters a state of hypersensitization.

This turns the brain into a "chemical trap" of permanent desire.

3.3 Tolerance, abstinence, and neuroadaptation

3.3.1 Tolerance: the Trick of Repetition

More substance is needed to achieve the same effect. There is pharmacological tolerance (desensitized receptors) and behavioral tolerance (associated routine).

Abstinence: the punishment of absence. It appears when use ceases. Symptoms may include:

- Physical: sweating, nausea, chills, and seizures.

- Psychic: dysphoria, nightmares, anxiety and obsessive thinking.

"I didn't use it to feel pleasure. I used it so as not to feel the hell of being unused".

3.3.2 Neuroadaptation: the New Pathological Balance

Over time:

- The endogenous production of dopamine, serotonin and GABA is reduced.
- Ion receptors and channels are modified.
- The brain reconfigures its basal state with substance as its axis.

This explains why recovery is not just about stopping using, but about retraining the brain.

3.4 Brain damage, Neuroinflammation, and Possible Recovery

3.4.1 Measurable Brain Damage

Neuroimaging has revealed:

- Cortical atrophy in the dorsolateral prefrontal cortex.
- Damage to white matter (communication routes).
- Decreased metabolism in the orbitofrontal cortex.

Areas such as the cerebellum, corpus callosum, and temporal lobes are also compromised in chronic users.

3.4.2 Chronic Neuroinflammation

Substances such as alcohol, cocaine, and methamphetamine cause:

- Activation of microglia → release of pro-inflammatory cytokines (IL-6, TNF-α).
- Damage to the blood-brain barrier.
- Sustained inflammatory epigenetic changes.

Neuroinflammation is related to anhedonia, post-use depression, and cognitive impairment. Is it reversible? Yes, but it depends on:

- substance used and duration,
- age of onset,
- medical and psychiatric comorbidities,
- social support and sustained treatment.

Neurogenesis in the **hippocampus and prefrontal** is possible with:

- aerobic exercise,
- meditation,
- occupational therapy,
- appropriate pharmacotherapy,
- Nutrition rich in omega 3, antioxidants and B vitamins.

3.5 Adolescence, Impulsivity and Neurodevelopment

3.5.1 The Adolescent Brain: a Construction Site

- **The prefrontal cortex** (reason, judgment) matures until the age of 24-25.
- **The limbic system** (emotions, pleasure) is activated earlier.
- Result: **car with a strong engine and weak brakes**.

This imbalance explains:

- Greater propensity to risk behaviors.
- Less sensitivity to punishment.

High vulnerability to developing long-lasting addiction if it begins before the age of 18.

1- Impact of Early Use

- Changes in **cerebral myelination**.
- Impaired working memory.
- Inhibition of emotional learning.
- Increased risk of developing BPD, ADHD, and affective disorders in young adults.

A week of cannabis use in an adolescent can alter the prefrontal cortex for 6 months.

3.6 Final Thoughts

The addicted brain is not simply a diseased **brain. It is a brain that learned to survive as best it could**, using what it had at its disposal.

The neuroscience of addiction does not seek to justify use, but to **understand the urgency and necessity behind each relapse**, **the biological trap that perpetuates consumption**, and **the long but possible road to repair**.

CHAPTER 4
Drugs that Trap: Classification and Effects. From the Classic to the Modern: Each Substance and its Trap

4.1 Alcohol

4.1.1 The Most Dangerous Legal Substance

Ethyl alcohol or ethanol is one of the most consumed psychoactive substances in the world. Although legal, it is responsible for more than 3 million deaths annually, according to the WHO. It is present in culture, ritual, leisure and suffering. Its use ranges from socially accepted to severe physical dependence with multisystemic impairment (Figure 4).

4.1.2 Types of Alcoholic Beverages

Category	Examples	Approximate Concentration
Fermented	Beer, wine, cider	3–14 %
Spirits	Vodka, whisky, ron, tequila	35–50 %
Liqueurs and mixed spirits	Amaretto, appetizers	15–30 %

A **standard unit** of alcohol is equivalent to:
- 330 ml of beer.
- 150 ml of wine.
- 45 ml of distilled liqueur.

4.1.3 Alcohol Pharmacology

- Rapid absorption by gastric and intestinal mucosa.
- Plasma peak in 30–90 min.

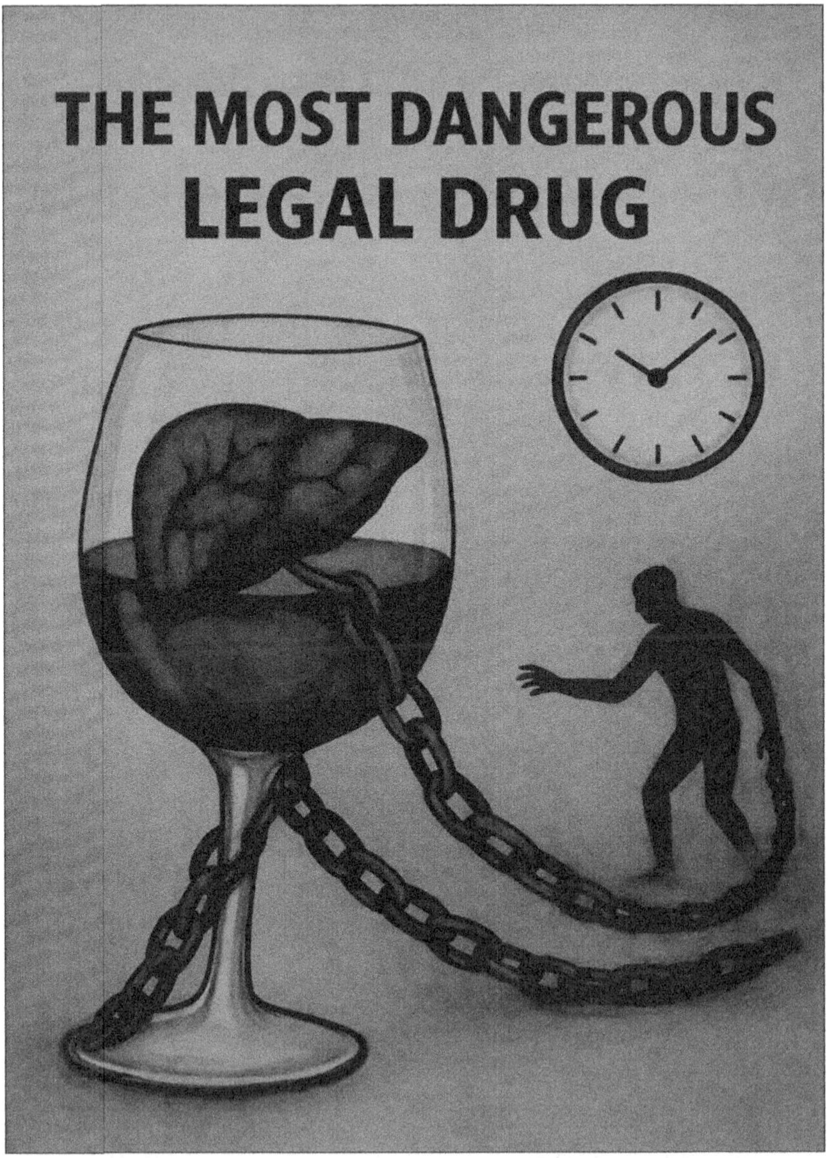

Figure 4. The most dangerous legal drug. This image symbolically represents the impact of alcohol as a legal, but highly destructive substance. The cup contains a chained liver, alluding to liver damage and the progressive dependence caused by alcohol. The chained human figure reflects the loss of freedom that addiction generates, while the clock suggests that deterioration is progressive and inevitable over time. A visual warning about the physical and existential toll of chronic alcohol use.

- Hepatic metabolism: alcohol dehydrogenase (ADH) → acetaldehyde (toxic) → acetate.

- Inhibition of NMDA receptors and potentiation of GABA-A.

- Affects dopamine, serotonin, endorphins, and the endogenous opioid system.

4.1.4 Short-term Effects by Dose

Dosage (g/l) approx.	Effects
0,2–0,5	Disinhibition, mild euphoria
0,5–1,5	Slurred language, clumsiness
1,5–3,0	Vomiting, incoherence, falls
> 3.0	Ethyl coma, bradipnea
> 4.0	Death from respiratory depression

4.1.5 Chronic Effects and Multi-organ Damage Brain

- Frontal cortical and cerebellar atrophy.

- Cognitive impairment (Korsakoff syndrome, Wernicke's encephalopathy).

- Depression, anxiety, alcoholic psychosis.

Liver

- Hepatic steatosis.

- Alcoholic hepatitis.

- Cirrosis (irreversible).

Heart

- Dilated cardiomyopathy.

- Arrhythmias.

- Hypertension.

Gastrointestinal tract

- Gastritis, ulcers, esophagitis.

- Cancer of the esophagus, liver, pancreas.

4.1.6 Fetal Alcohol Spectrum Disorders (FASDs)

Alcohol use in pregnancy can cause:

- Microcephaly.
- Abnormal facial features.
- Cognitive and developmental delay.
- Learning disorders.

There is no "safe amount" of alcohol during pregnancy.

4.1.7 Diagnosis of Alcohol Dependence Clinical Criteria (DSM-5)

- Persistent desire to drink.
- Failure to reduce.
- Use despite the damage.
- Tolerance and abstinence.
- A lot of time dedicated to consumption.

Useful tools:

- Alcohol Use Disorders Identification Test (AUDIT).
- Cut-down, Annoyed, Guilty, Eye-opener (CAGE).

4.1.8 Alcohol Use Disorder Identification Test (AUDIT)

What is it?

The **AUDIT** is a 10-question questionnaire developed by the WHO to detect risky, harmful or dependent consumption of alcohol.

Structure:

It is divided into 3 areas:

- Questions 1–3: Alcohol use (frequency and quantity).
- Questions 4–6: Symptoms of dependence.
- Questions 7–10: Consequences or harms related to consumption.

Each question is graded from **0 to 4 points**, and the total score ranges from **0 to 40**.

Interpretation:
- 0–7 points: Low-risk consumption.
- 8–15 points: Risky consumption.
- 16–19 points: Harmful consumption.
- 20 or more: Probable alcohol dependence.

4.1.9 Examples (selected questions):

Q1. How often do you drink any alcoholic beverages?

Never (0), Less than 1 time/month (1), 2–4 times/month (2), 2–3 times/week (3), 4 or more times/week (4).

Example: "I drink wine 3 times a week" → Score: 3

Q3. How often do you have 6 or more alcoholic drinks at one time?

Example: "Every Friday I drink like 7 beers" → Score: 3

Q4. How often in the past year have you been unable to stop drinking once you started?

Example: "Sometimes I start and don't stop until I finish the bottle" → Score: 2

Q9. Have you or anyone else been injured due to your alcohol consumption?

Example: "I once fell and hit my head after drinking" → Score: 2

4.1.10 CAGE Questionnaire

What is it?

The **CAGE** is a very short **4-question questionnaire**, ideal for quick medical consultations. It is used to detect possible **problems with alcohol at any time of life**. The name is an acronym in English:

C (Cutdown): Have you felt like you need to cut back on your drinking?

A (Annoyed): Have you been bothered by others criticizing your drinking?

G (Guilty): Have you felt guilty about your drinking?

E (Eye-opener): Have you ever needed to drink alcohol in the morning to feel better (as an alarm clock)?

Interpretation:

2 yes or more answers → High suspicion of alcohol use disorder.

Examples:

C–Cutdown

"My wife tells me I should drink less, and I've thought about it". → **Yes**

A–Annoyed

"My co-workers said I smell like beer in the mornings, and that bothered me". → **Yes**

G–Guilty

"I felt embarrassed for drinking on my son's birthday". → **Yes**

E–Eye-opener

"Sometimes I take a shot of vodka when I wake up to get rid of the tremors". → **Yes**

Comparative Summary

Tool	Format	Purpose	Time Evaluated	Ideal for
AUDIT	10 items with score	Detects risky consumption or dependence	Last 12 months	Clinics, public health
I screwed up	4 yes/no questions	Detects alcohol problems throughout life	Anytime	Quick consultations in medicine

4.1.11 Alcohol Withdrawal Syndrome

It occurs 6-24 h after the last dose in dependent patients.

Phase	Features
Mild	Tremors, anxiety, insomnia
Moderate	Hallucinations, tachycardia, sweating

Phase	Features
Delirium tremens	Confusion, fever, visual hallucinations, risk of death
Seizures	Generalized, tonic-clonic type

4.1.12 Treatment of Alcoholism

Acute phase (withdrawal)

Long-acting benzodiazepines:

1- Diazepam 10–20 mg every 6 h, adjust according to CIWA-Ar.

Supplementation of:

2- Thiamine IM: 100–300 mg/day (prevention of Wernicke).

3- Folic acid, magnesium.

4- Hydration, BP monitoring, heart monitor.

Maintenance Phase (Relapse Prevention)

Medication	Dosage	Mechanism
Naltrexone oral	50 mg/day	Blocks the opioid system, reduces craving
Vivitrol (IM)	380 mg/month	Extended-release version
Acamprosato	666 mg TID	Modulates glutamate, reduces anxiety
Disulfiram	250–500 mg/day	Inhibits ALDH → aversive reaction

Disulfiram requires informed consent and strict medical supervision.

Psychotherapeutic interventions

- Cognitive behavioral therapy (CBT).
- Motivational interviewing.
- Relapse prevention therapy.

- Support groups (AA, SMART Recovery).
- Structured family intervention.

Clinical case

Juan, 46 years old, functional alcoholic. Drink 1 liter of rum daily, hide bottles in the office. When he leaves it, he suffers convulsions and hallucinations. He was hospitalized 3 times. After starting naltrexone and intensive therapy, she achieved 6 months of abstinence.

4.2 Tobacco and Nicotine

4.2.1 The Silent Addiction that Breathes, Hides and Kills

Tobacco is the leading cause of preventable death worldwide. According to the World Health Organization:

- More than 8 million people die each year as a result of tobacco.
- 1.3 million of those deaths are due to exposure to second-hand smoke.
- Each cigarette shortens a person's life by an average of 11 minutes.

Nicotine, its main active component, is one of the most addictive substances that exist, due to:

- Rapid onset (reaches the brain in 10 seconds).
- Short duration of action (30-40 minutes).
- High frequency of reinforcement (1 cigar = 10-15 puffs).

4.2.2 Forms of Consumption

Method	Description
Cigarette	The most common, highly processed, with dozens of additives
Pure/Tobacco	Slow burning, higher nicotine concentration

Method	Description
Pipe	Common in rituals; alkaline smoke; Risk of oral cancer
Chewing tobacco/snuff	Absorbed by oral or nasal mucosa; High oral damage
Snus (Swedish style)	It is placed on the upper gum; Less harmful than smoking
Vaporizers/e-cigs	Nicotine aerosolized with flavorings; Growing use in teens

A teenager who uses one vape cartridge a day may be absorbing the equivalent of 1-2 packs of cigarettes.

4.2.3 Nicotine Pharmacodynamics

Nicotine stimulates nicotinic acetylcholine receptors (nAChRs) in the brain and autonomic nervous system.

Main neurochemical effects:

- **Dopamine (nucleus accumbens): reward, longing.**
- **Noradrenaline:** increased attention and blood pressure.
- **Serotonin:** transient regulation of mood.
- **Endorphins:** brief feeling of well-being.
- **Adrenaline:** tachycardia, vasoconstriction.

It acts in seconds and disappears in 30-60 minutes, causing rapid cycles of desire.

4.2.4 Factors that Increase the Risk of Addiction

- Early onset (< 18 years).
- Priests or caregivers, smokers.
- Comorbidities such as ADHD, anxiety, depression.
- Media normalization (influencers, movies, music).
- Mistaken belief that vaping is "safe" or "harmless".

4.2.5 Immediate Effects

System	Effects
Brain	Mild euphoria, increased focus
Heart	Increased heart rate and pressure
Digestive	Appetite suppression, mild nausea
Lungs	Bronchial irritation, initial cough
Encouragement	Rebound anxiety 30 minutes after smoking

Clinical Testimony

"I feel calm when I smoke, but if I can't, I feel like I'm losing control" (29-year-old smoker with untreated anxiety).

4.2.6 Long-term Multisystem Damage

Pulmonary

- Chronic bronchitis.
- Emphysema.
- Chronic obstructive pulmonary disease.
- Lung cancer (90% linked to tobacco).

Cardiovascular

- Increased coagulation and blood viscosity.
- Accelerated atherosclerosis.
- Myocardial infarctions and stroke.
- Aortic aneurysms.

Cancer risk

Tobacco smoke contains more than 70 known carcinogens.

Site	Relative Risk (Smoker versus Nonsmoker)
Lungs	20-30 times
Esophagus	10-15 times
Mouth/Larynx	8-20 times
Bladder/kidney	5-7 times
Pancreas/stomach	times

4.2.7 Risks in Pregnancy and Childhood

- Low birth weight.
- Abortion, premature birth.
- Sudden infant death syndrome.
- Increased risk of asthma, obesity, and ADHD in children (Figure 5).

4.2.8 Auge of the Vapeo

Truths about e-cigarettes:

- They contain highly concentrated nicotine salts.
- They are usually combined with diacetyl, propylene glycol, and heavy metals.
- They generate aerosolized microtoxins that penetrate deep into the lungs.
- Linked to vaping-associated lung injury (EVALI).

One in four teens who vape also use cannabis or drugs.

4.2.9 Diagnosis of Nicotine Use Disorder

Clinical indicators:

- Smoking/vaping within the first 30 minutes of waking up.
- Failed attempts to quit.

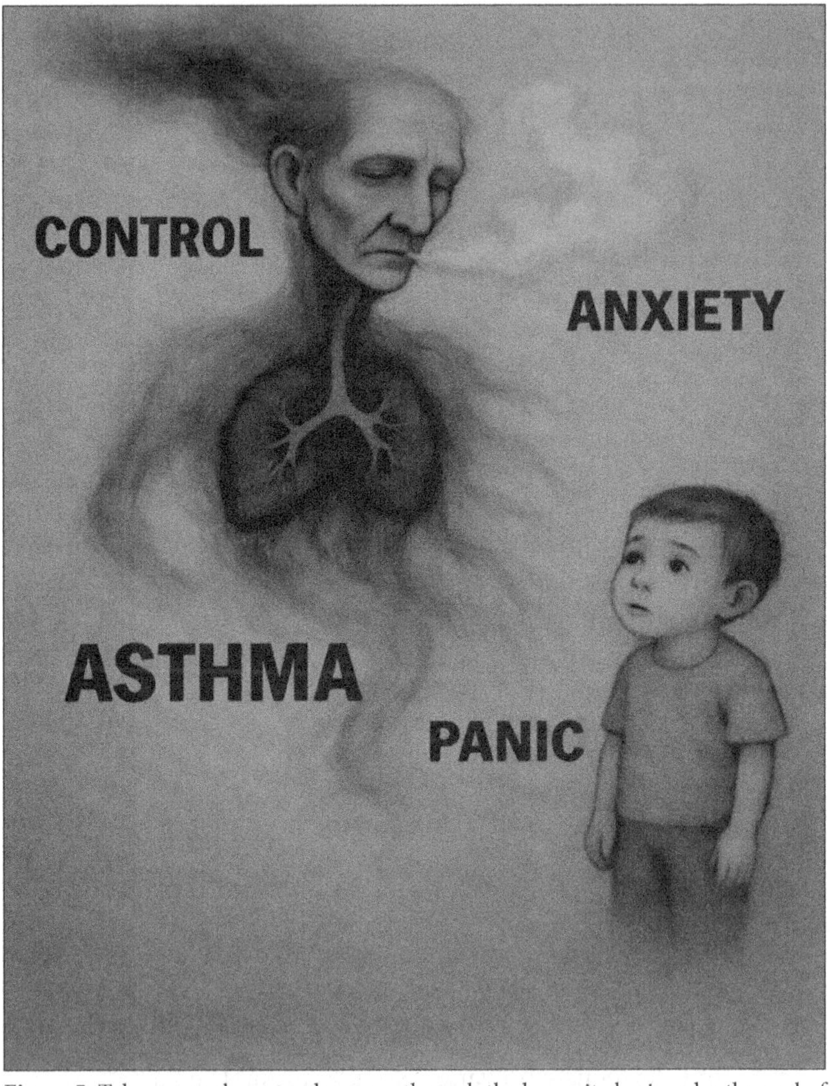

Figure 5. Tobacco smoke not only passes through the lungs, it also invades the soul of the child who observes. This image depicts how anxiety, asthma, the desire for control, and panic are passed down from generation to generation, leaving invisible but profound imprints on the emotional and respiratory health of the children of smokers.

- Withdrawal symptoms.
- Continued use despite health problems.

Use the Fagerström Test to assess dependence.

4.2.10 Nicotine Withdrawal Syndrome

Symptom	Spawn Time	Duration
Anxiety/irritability	2-6 hours	1-3 weeks
Insomnia	1-3 days	Up to 4 weeks
Low mood	1-2 days	Up to 6 weeks
Increased appetite	2-4 days	1-3 months
Craving	Constant	Can last for months

Clinical Testimony

"I dream that I smoke. When I wake up and I can't do it, I feel desperate" (patient in withdrawal).

4.2.11 Omprehensive Treatment

Brief intervention (in any clinical setting):

- "Have you thought about quitting?"
- "How many cigarettes do you smoke a day?"
- "What would happen if you quit smoking today?"

A short intervention of just three minutes can increase the dropout rate by 30-50%.

4.2.12 Pharmacological Treatment

Treatment	Starting dose	Mechanism
Varenicline	0.5 mg → 1 mg BID	nAChR partial agonist
Bupropion SR	150 mg → 300 mg/day	DA/NE Recapture Inhibitor
Nicotine patches	7 / 14 / 21 mg/day	Slow and continuous release
Rubber/Tablets/Spray	2–4 mg every 1–2 h	Quick Relief from Craving

The combination of nicotine replacement therapy (NRT) + oral medication offers the highest success rate (up to 60%).

4.2.13 Psychological Support

- CBT focused on triggers and emotional regulation.
- Strategies for weight management.
- Group therapy and family engagement.
- Mobile apps and text messaging.
- Relapse prevention planning.

Clinical case

Adriana, 38, started smoking at 14. He tried to quit 9 times. His partner also smokes, which makes it more difficult. He has palpitations and anxiety. With bupropion + NRT + CBT, he has not smoked for four months. She required psychiatric follow-up for anxiety.

4.3 Marijuana and Cannabinoids

The plant that calms the body, rests the mind and captures the will. Natural... but not harmless. Marijuana, also known as cannabis, weed, weed or ganja, is the **most widely used illegal psychoactive drug in the world**, although its legal status is changing in many regions.

Although it has been revered for its spiritual and medicinal uses, its use is also associated with **addiction**, **psychiatric instability**, and **cognitive impairment**, especially in adolescents and people with genetic vulnerability (Figure 6).

According to the CDC, about **30% of frequent users develop cannabis use disorder**, and the risk increases with early onset, frequency, and use of products with a high concentration of tetrahydrocannabinol (THC), the main psychoactive compound in cannabis that alters the mind and produces effects such as euphoria and relaxation.

4.3.1 Chemical Composition and Cannabis Strains

Cannabis contains more than **100 phytocannabinoids**, of which the most well-known are those shown in the table below:

Component	Main Effect and Action
THC	Tetrahydrocannabinol; main psychoactive; causes euphoria, altered perception, and appetite stimulation
CBD	Cannabidiol; non-psychoactive; anxiolytic, anti-inflammatory, anticonvulsant
CBG, CBN, CBC	Minor cannabinoids under study: mood modulation and inflammation

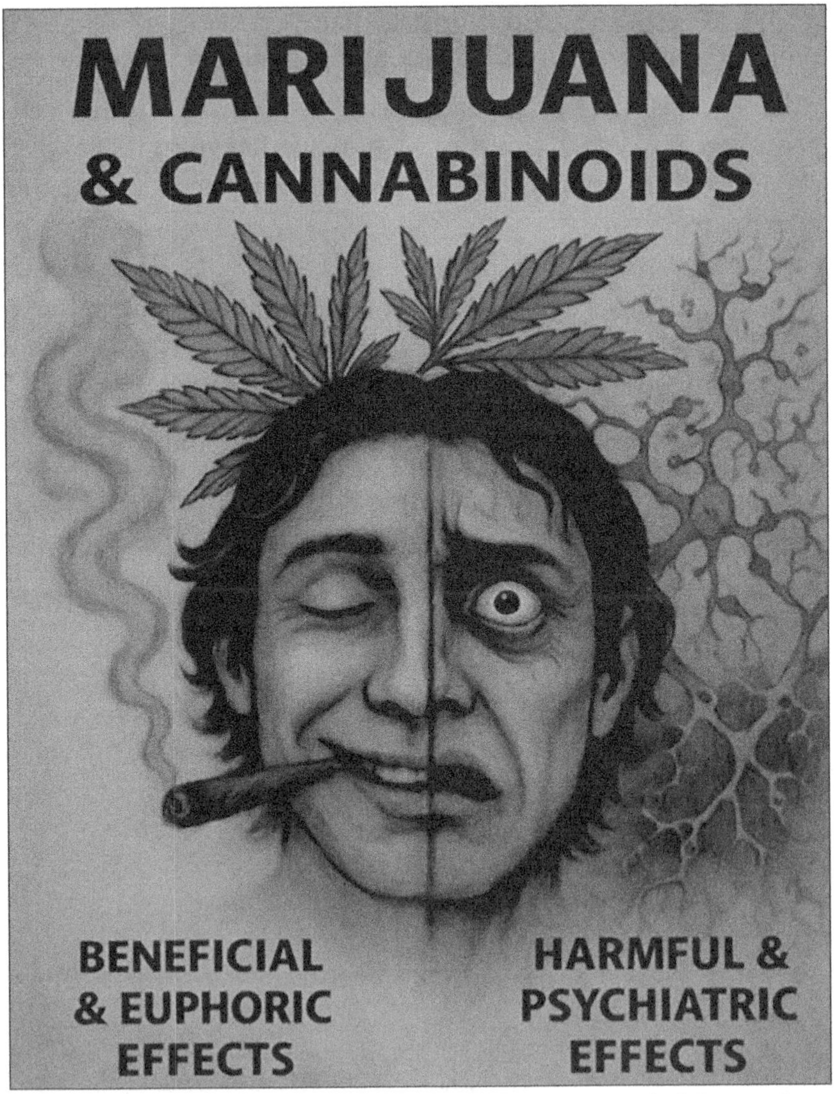

Figure 6. The illustration depicts the double face of marijuana: on the left, its euphoric and pleasurable effects; on the right, the negative consequences at the cerebral and psychiatric level. The leaves as a crown evoke his naturalness, while the split face reveals the ambivalence of his impact on the human being.

4.3.2 Types of cannabis

Variety	Common Effects
Sativa	Stimulating, euphoric, more cerebral; can induce anxiety
Indica	Sedative, body relaxing, physical effects
Hybrid	Variable mixing of both features

Modern strains can contain **up to 10 times more** THC than those of 30 years ago due to genetic modifications and concentrate extraction.

4.3.3 Forms of Consumption and their Clinical Implications

Route of Use	Home	Duration	Clinical Risks
Smoked/vaped	2-5 min	1-3 hrs	Immediate effect; Inhalation of tar and toxins
Groceries	30-90 min	4-8 hrs	Increased risk of overdose due to delayed effect
Concentrates (dabs, wax, shatter)	1-2 min	2-4 hrs	THC >70%; High risk of psychosis
Sublingual/Accepted	15-45 min	2-6 hrs	More controlled dose; Therapeutic Use

A single brownie can have more THC than 10 ordinary joints.

4.3.4 Mechanism of Action: the Endocannabinoid System

THC acts on the **CB1** (brain) and **CB2** (immune) receptors, part of the endocannabinoid system (ECS), which regulates:

- mood,
- pain,

- sleep,
- memory,
- appetite,
- inflammation.

Receptor	Location	Main Function
CB1	Cortex, amygdala, hippocampus	Memory, pleasure, emotions, coordination
CB2	Immune cells and peripheral tissues	Regulation of inflammation

THC **mimics anandamide**, but with more intense and long-lasting effects, which disrupts brain homeostasis.

4.3.5 Acute Effects: between Euphoria and Dysphoria

Most common effects:
- euphoria, spontaneous laughter,
- alteration of time and space,
- sensory stimulation (food, music, colors),
- increased appetite,
- immediate memory disorders,
- anxiety or paranoia, especially in high doses.

Clinical Testimony

"At first I felt enlightened. Then I thought they were reading my mind" (24-year-old frequent user).

4.3.6 Long-term Effects

Cognitive impairment:
- less sustained attention,

- reduction of working memory,
- difficulty in verbal learning,
- loss of motivation.

Longitudinal studies show a loss of up to 8 IQ points in chronic users who started before the age of 18.

4.3.7 Emotional and Psychiatric Impact

Disorder	Relevant Clinical Notes
Cannabis-induced psychosis	Hallucinations, paranoia, delusions.
Generalized anxiety or panic attacks	It can be caused by THC.
Depression	Frequent in prolonged use.
Bipolarity	Destabilization of phases; increased irritability.
Schizophrenia	4-7 times higher risk in vulnerable young people.

In people with a genetic predisposition, cannabis can trigger a first psychotic break (Figure 7).

Motivational syndrome:
- apathy,
- social retreat,
- loss of goals,
- lack of personal interest.

Clinical Testimony

"I used to compose songs. Now I spend the day watching TikTok" (19-year-old chronic user).

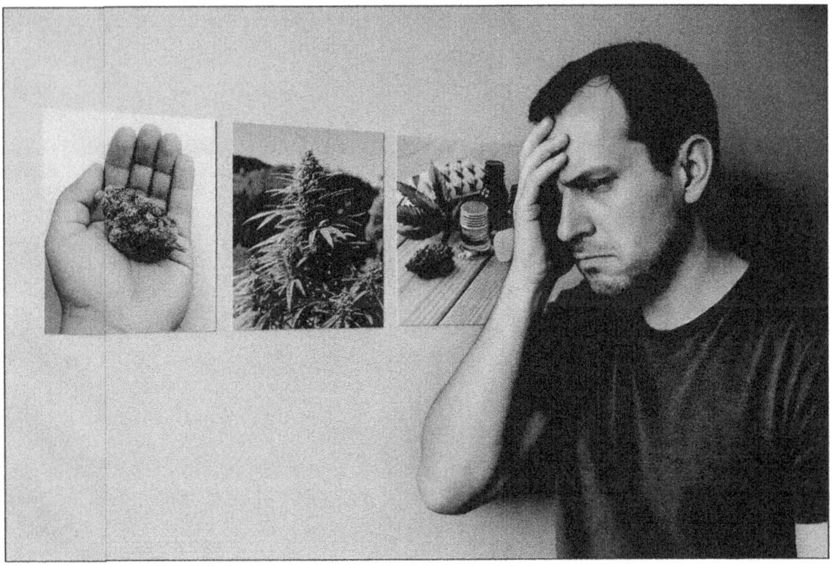

Figure 7. A distraught man looks at images of marijuana in its various forms: natural, grown, and processed. The scene depicts the internal conflict of those dealing with cannabis addiction, between the perception of naturalness and the adverse emotional effects that can arise with prolonged use.

4.3.8 Dependence and Abstinence

Dependence (cannabis use disorder)

- Appears in ~10% of users.
- Up to 30% in those who consume daily.
- In teens, it may be 1 in 6.

Withdrawal syndrome

Symptom	Home	Duration
Irritability	Day 1–3	Up to 2 weeks
Insomnia	Day 2–4	2–4 weeks
Vivid nightmares	Day 3–5	1–2 weeks
Anxiety and craving	Variable	Months

4.3.9 Medical Cannabis: Real Uses and Risks

Uses with moderate to strong evidence:

- Refractory neuropathic pain.
- Spasticity in multiple sclerosis.
- Nausea due to chemotherapy.
- Severe epilepsies in children (pure CBD).

Risks:

- Homemade products without dosage.
- Young people with anxiety → risk of addiction.
- Therapeutic justification without formal medical indication.

Clinical Testimony

"I started using CBD for sleep. I ended up vaping THC every day" (31-year-old woman).

4.3.10 Synthetic Cannabinoids: "The chemist", Spice, K2

They are artificial compounds, not derived from the plant, more potent and less predictable.

Effects:

- Acute psychosis.
- Aggressiveness, tachycardia, seizures.
- Not detectable in standard urine tests.

A single dose can lead to emergency psychiatric hospitalization.

4.3.11 Cannabis Use Disorder Treatment

Effective psychotherapies:

- Cognitive behavioral therapy (CBT).
- Motivational interview.
- contingency management.
- structured family therapy (youth).

Drugs under study (not officially approved):

- ISRS (fluoxetine, sertraline).
- Gabapentina.
- Quetiapina.
- N-acetylcysteine (antioxidant with craving regulating effect).

Clinical cases

Clinical case 1. Functional Consumption

Carlos, 17 years old. He smoked since he was 14. His school performance dropped, he stopped sports. He said: "weed relaxes me". When he tried to quit, he suffered insomnia, night sweats and anxiety. Diagnosis: moderate cannabis use disorder.

Clinical case 2. Psychosis

Adriana, 26 years old, daily user of dabs. He began to hear voices and have paranoid ideas. Family history of schizophrenia. He was admitted with induced psychosis. He improved after stopping THC and antipsychotic treatment.

4.4 Cocaine and Crack Cocaine

4.4.1 From Andean Ritual to Urban Collapse

Cocaine comes from the coca leaf, used ancestrally by indigenous peoples of the Andes for ritual, energy and sacred purposes. However, the industrial refinement of the alkaloid and its illegal commercialization transformed this plant into **one of the most addictive, destructive and trafficked drugs in the world**.

According to the United Nations Office on Drugs and Crime (UNODC), more than **22 million people** use cocaine annually. It is the drug of **extremes**: glamour and misery, energy and devastation, power and ruin.

4.4.2 Types, Street Names and Forms of Consumption

Substance	Street Name	Route of Use	Clinical Comments
Powder Cocaine	Perico, pass, yeyo, farlopa, snow	Sniffed, injected	Brief euphoria; risk of nasal necrosis and overdose.
Crack	Stone, Base, Rock	Smoked in a pipe or bottle	Intense euphoria for 5-10 min; high pulmonary toxicity.
Basuco/ paco	Cheap crack residues	Smoked with a rag or paper	Very impure; used in street populations.

It can be mixed with other drugs: speedball (cocaine + heroin), which increases the risk of sudden death.

4.4.3 Neurobiology: The Synaptic Storm

Cocaine is a **potent inhibitor of the reuptake of dopamine, norepinephrine and serotonin**. This causes accumulation in the synaptic cleft, especially in the **mesolimbic system** (nucleus accumbens, ventral tegmental area).

What happens in the brain:

- **Dopamine:** hyperpleasure → addictive reinforcement → subsequent anhedonia.
- **Noradrenaline:** extreme alert → tachycardia, hypertension.
- **Serotonin:** sexual disinhibition → irritability and post-use dysphoria.

Cocaine **destroys the dopaminergic balance**, and the brain is left underfunctioning without it → depression, irritability and craving.

4.4.4 Sharp Effects (Minute by Minute)

Minute	Sensation
0-2	Euphoric peak, feeling of total power
3-15	Hyperactivity, verbiage, elevated libido
15-30	Irritability, muscle tension, sweating
30-60	Onset of downturn: anxiety, mild paranoia
>60	Intense craving: compulsive desire to repeat

Crack has a more violent onset and a steeper fall. This generates a **chain consumption** every 10-15 minutes.

4.4.5 Medium and Long-term Medical Consequences

Neurological and psychiatric:

- Cocaine psychosis: persecutory delusions, tactile hallucinations ("bugs under the skin").
- Extreme paranoia, violent impulsivity.
- Elevated risk of suicide in the downturn.

Cardiovascular:

- Acute myocardial infarction (in young people).
- Ventricular arrhythmias.
- Malignant hypertension.
- Fulminant aortic dissection.

Respiratory (crack, paco):

- Bronchospasm.
- Spontaneous pneumothorax.

- "Crack lung" (chemical alveolitis).
- Chronic cough, blackish cough.

Digestive and NCDs:

- Nasal perforation (due to chronic snorting).
- Mouth ulcers and gastritis.
- Hepatitis and HIV from shared syringes.

4.4.6 Addictive Cycle and Compulsive Behavior

The pattern of use generates a vicious circle:

- **Craving:** fixed thought on consuming.
- **Use:** Powerful dose → hyperpleasure.
- **Downside:** dysphoria, guilt, insomnia.
- **Rebound:** more craving→ continuous use.
- **Burnout:** permanent anxiety, paranoia and isolation.

Clinical Testimony

"I consume 10 stones a night. When I don't have any, I'm afraid even of my children. I feel that people follow me" (homeless man, 36 years old).

4.4.7 The World of Crack: Marginality, Prison and Death

Crack has devastated poor urban areas. It's cheap, powerful, and easy to make. Smoking in:

- Broken bottles.
- Improvised pipes with metal, aluminum and plastic.
- Soaked rags ("el fierrito").

Social consequences:

- Prostitution by dose.
- Children who smoke from 9–10 years old.
- Robbery, violence, family abandonment.

Severe lung infections, TB, HIV.

4.4.8 Abstinence and Craving

Phase	Duration	Symptoms
Phase 1 (Crash)	24–72 hrs	Extreme fatigue, depression, anhedonia
Phase 2 (Retirement)	Weeks	Irritability, insomnia, anxiety, intense dreams
Phase 3 (Extinction)	Months	Intermittent craving , triggered by environmental cues

Unlike alcohol or BZD, **cocaine withdrawal is not medical, but emotionally and mentally devastating** (Figure 8).

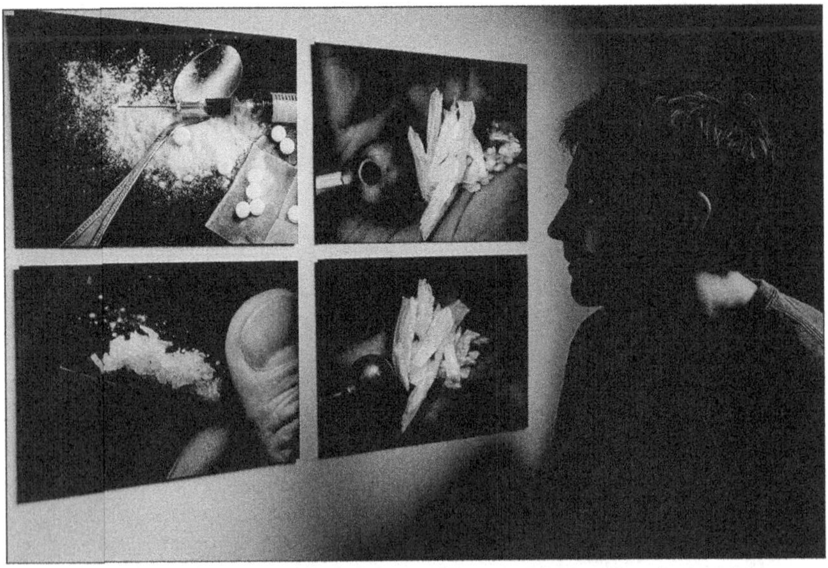

Figure 8. A man silently contemplates several images of stimulant drugs: white powder, methamphetamine crystals and crack pipes. His tense face reflects the weight of compulsion. This scene illustrates the initial magnetism of cocaine and crack, which contrasts with the progressive devastation of the body and mind.

4.4.9 Treatment of Cocaine and Crack Use Disorder

Acute intervention:

- Benzodiacepinas (lorazepam 2-4 mg).
- Atypical antipsychotics if delusions are present (olanzapine 5-10 mg).
- IV serum, BP and ECG control.
- Observation for risk of aggression or suicide.

4.4.10 Maintenance Therapies

Therapy/Drug	Clinical Objective
Cognitive behavioral therapy (CBT)	Restructure addictive thoughts and behaviors
Contingency Management	Documented abstinence rewards
Group therapy	NA, CA, therapeutic communities
N-acetylcysteine	Glutamatergic modulator → reduces craving
Bupropion/topiramate	Boost reduction and craving
Disulfiram (experimental)	Peripheral dopaminergic inhibition

The key is the **intensive**, **prolonged approach with multiple simultaneous pillars.**

Clinical cases

Clinical case 1. Functional Executive

Andrés, 38 years old, bank manager. He began to "snort to work harder". He ends up consuming daily, loses control, steals money to buy. When he was hospitalized, he admits: "I became a monster with a tie".

Clinical case 2. Street Addiction

Mayra, 21 years old. She lives in a vacant lot, mother of a baby, smokes paco with aluminum foil. Malnutrition, active TB, severe lung lesions. She was admitted to a center for pregnant women with psychiatric support and social work (Figure 9).

4.5 Amphetamines and Methamphetamine

Artificial energy, real destruction: from extreme performance to devastating psychosis. Amphetamines and methamphetamine are potent stimulants of the central nervous system (CNS). Although some versions are used therapeutically (such as in the treatment of ADHD or narcolepsy), their recreational and street use has given rise to one of the most dangerous, rapidly deteriorating and psychiatrically charged addictions (Figure 10).

4.5.1 Types, Street Names, and Presentations

Substance	Street Names	Presentation	Management Path
Amphetamines	Speed, pills, tablets	Tablets, capsules	Oral, inhaled, injected
Methamphetamine	Crystal, stone, meth, ice	Crystals, dust	Smoked, inhaled, IV
Bath salts (synthetic cathinones)	Flakka, MDPV, etc.	Synthetic powders	Inhalation, smoked

Pharmaceutical forms such as **Adderall** (amphetamine-dextroamphetamine) and **Desoxyn** (medical methamphetamine) can be legally used by prescription, but abuse is common.

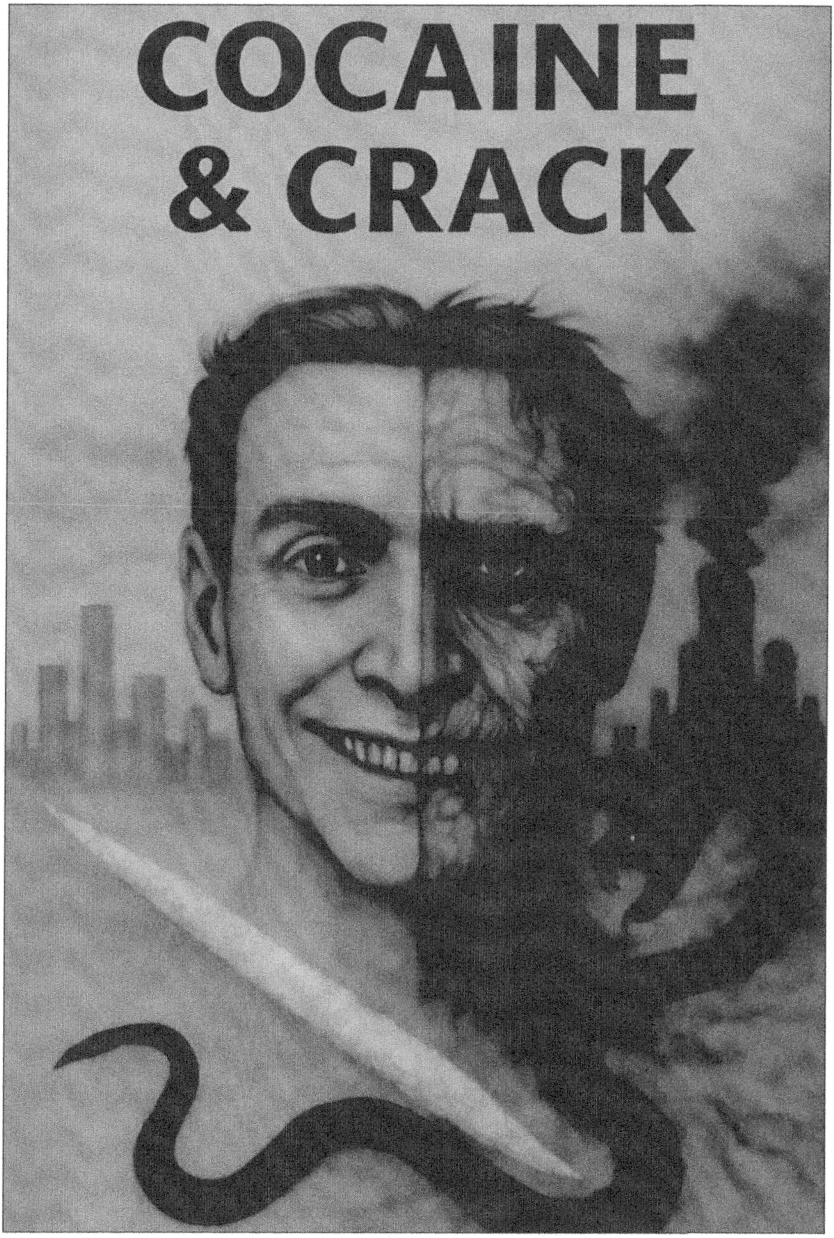

Figure 9. A symbolic portrait of the decline in cocaine and crack: a face divided between initial euphoria and final deterioration. The snaking white line turns into a venomous snake, reflecting how fleeting pleasure leads to physical, emotional, and social destruction.

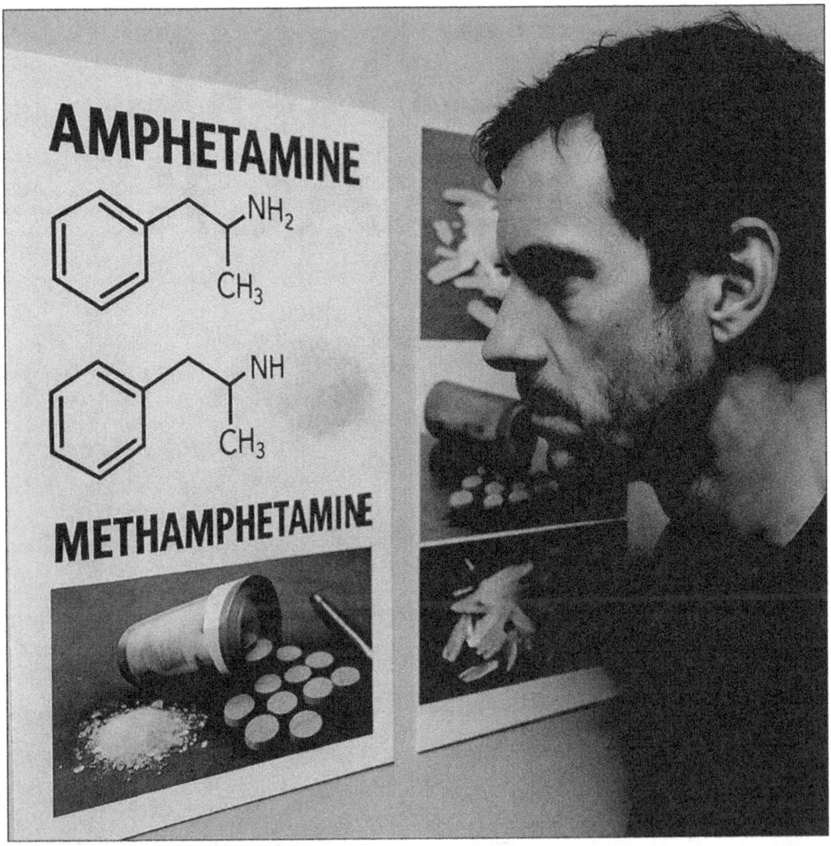

Figure 10. A man looks with concern at posters showing the chemical structures and pharmaceutical and street presentations of amphetamines and methamphetamine, reflecting the bridge between medical use and devastating abuse.

4.5.2 Mechanism of Action: Extreme Neurostimulation

Amphetamines and methamphetamine increase the release and block the reuptake of dopamine, norepinephrine, and serotonin, causing an excessive buildup of these neurotransmitters in the brain. Methamphetamine crosses the blood-brain barrier more quickly and acts with a prolonged intensity, which can last up to 12 hours.

4.5.3 Immediate Effects of Consumption

Area	Typical Effects
Mental	Euphoria, hyperactivity, verbiage, increased confidence
Physical	Tachycardia, dilated pupils, decreased appetite
Sexual	Increased desire and impulsive behavior (chemsex)
Cognitive	Feeling of clarity, concentration, productivity
Mood	Irritability, insomnia, progressive aggression

Clinical Testimony

"I worked 72 hours straight without stopping or eating. In the end I thought the FBI was spying on me" (27-year-old programmer, methamphetamine user).

4.5.4 Long-term Use: Physical and Psychiatric Effects

4.5.4.1 Physical Effects

- "Meth mouth": severe cavities, tooth loss, receding gums.
- Extreme weight loss.
- Skin lesions from compulsive scratching.
- Premature aging.
- Chronic insomnia

4.5.4.2 Psychiatric Effects:

- Persistent paranoid psychosis.
- Visual, auditory, and tactile hallucinations.
- Delusions of persecution.
- Mood disorders.

Methamphetamine-induced psychosis can persist weeks after withdrawal.

4.5.5 Neurocognitive Impact

- Reduced brain volume in key areas such as the prefrontal cortex and hippocampus.
- Deficits in working memory, sustained attention and decision-making.
- Impairment of executive functions.
- Permanent mood disorders.

Neuroimaging studies have shown a significant decrease in the density of dopamine transporters in chronic methamphetamine users.

4.5.6 Associated Behaviors

- Chemsex: sexualized consumption with multiple partners and without protection.
- Methamphetamine "Runs": 2-5 days without sleep, with compulsive use.
- Elevated risk of HIV, hepatitis, and other sexually transmitted diseases (STDs).
- Criminal and aggressive behavior.

Clinical Testimony

"I was convinced that there were microphones in my kitchen lamp" (32-year-old woman, with a psychotic break due to meth).

4.5.7 Abstinence and Craving

Withdrawal syndrome:

- Anhedonia severa.
- Extreme fatigue.
- Prolonged sleep (hypersomnia).
- Anxiety and agitation.
- Suicidal ideation.
- Persistent craving.

Abstinence can last from 1 to 3 weeks, with psychological craving persisting for months.

4.5.8 Comprehensive Treatment

4.5.8.1 Psychiatric Emergencies

- Antipsychotics (olanzapine, risperidone).
- Benzodiazepines (lorazepam) for severe agitation.
- Hydration, containment and observation for 24-72 hours.

4.5.8.2 Psychotherapy

- Cognitive behavioral therapy (CBT).
- Contingency therapy (abstinence rewards).
- Structured recovery groups.
- Intensive motivational approach.

4.5.9 Pharmacotherapy under Study

There are currently no approved drug treatments specifically for methamphetamine use disorder. However, recent studies have explored the combined use of extended-release naltrexone and bupropion, showing promising results in reducing consumption.

Clinical cases

Clinical case 1. Destructive "Functionality"

Sebastián, 35 years old, financial consultant. It started with Adderall. He migrated to methamphetamine to "perform better". Within two years, he lost his job, lost his partner, and was hospitalized for a psychotic break with satellite control ideas.

Clinical case 2. Sexualized Consumption

Luis, 29 years old, HIV positive. He participated in parties with meth and unprotected sex for 3-5 days in a row. He presented visual hallucinations and aggressiveness. Treated with risperidone and containment in a psychiatric unit (Figure 11).

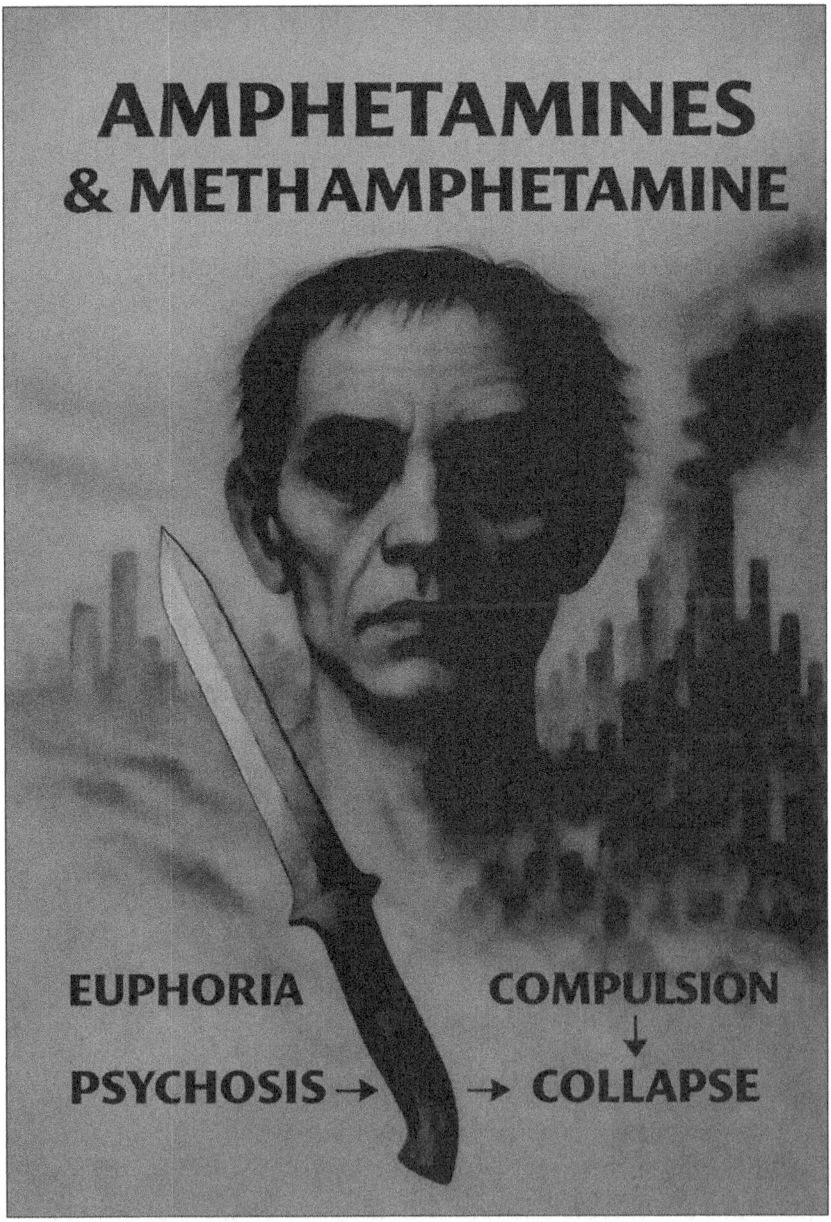

Figure 11. A dark portrait of the deterioration caused by amphetamines and methamphetamine: an emaciated face, a collapsed city in the background and a knife that symbolizes the journey from euphoria to psychosis, compulsion and total collapse.

4.6 Heroin, Fentanyl, and Opioids

4.6.1 The Promise of Relief... that Ends with the Breath

Opioids were born as balms for suffering. From Sumerian tablets to modern hospitals, their history is intertwined with medicine, war, spirituality, and the black market. But when pain becomes escape, opioids —no longer compassionate— trap, degrade, and silence (Figure 12).

In the United States, opioid overdoses kill more than 100 people a day. Fentanyl is now the leading cause of death among young adults.

4.6.2 General Classification of Opioids

Type of opioid	Examples	Approximate Potency with Respect to Morphine
Natural	Morphine, codeine	1x to 0.1x
Semi-synthetic	Heroin, oxycodone, hydromorphone	2x to 5x
Synthetics	Fentanyl, methadone, tramadol	50x (fentanyl) to 100x (carfentanil)

Did you know?

- Carfentanil is 10,000 times more potent than morphine. It was designed to immobilize elephants.

- A single poorly cut dose can cause respiratory arrest in seconds.

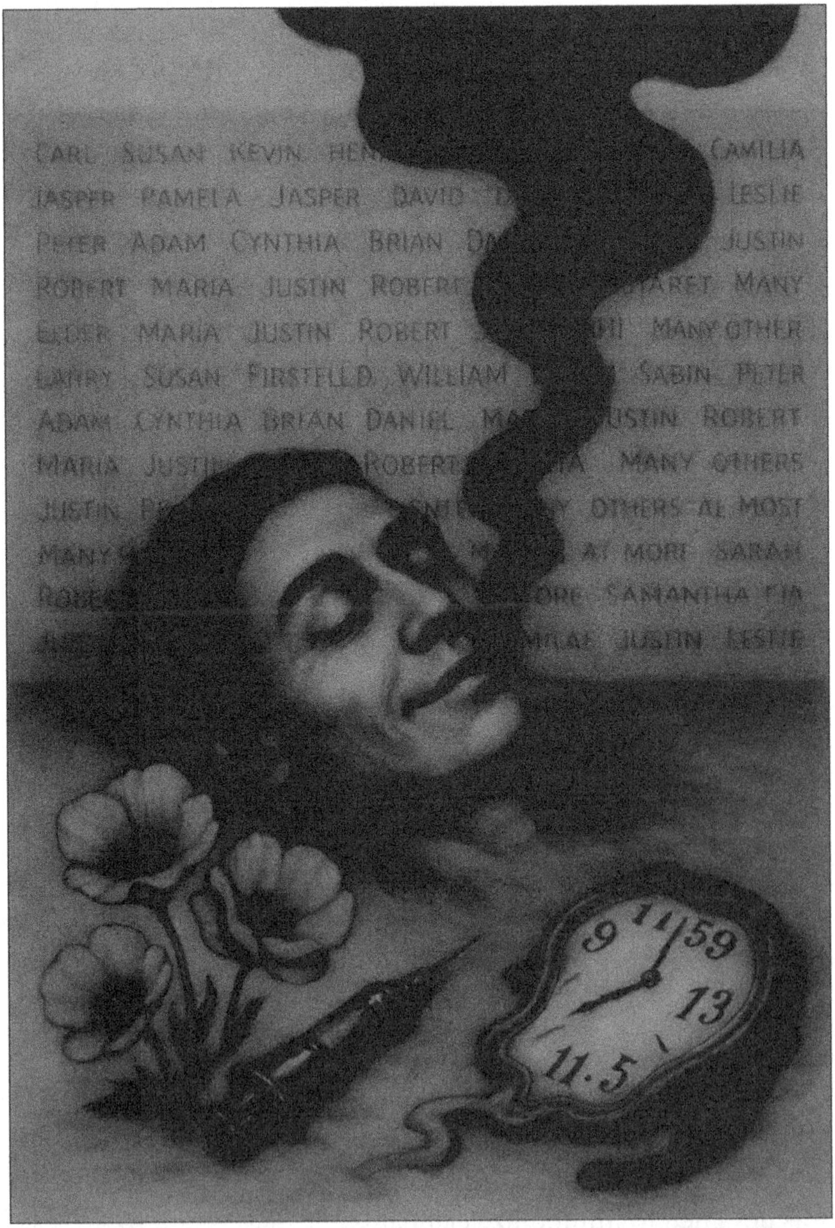

Figure 12. A symbolic image shows a man seemingly at peace as a cloud of opioids rises from his face, surrounded by poppies, a syringe and a melted clock —metaphors for relief, addiction and the passage of time to death. The names engraved in the background pay tribute to those who lost their lives to overdoses.

4.6.2.1 Administration Routes and Consumer Culture

Method	Drug Used	Cultural and Medical Description
Injected	Heroin, fentanyl	High bioavailability, risk of HIV/HCV
Inhaled	Heroin, fentanyl, oxy	"Chasingthedragon": aluminum foil and flame
Oral	Tramadol, oxicodona	Slower onset, but high dependency
Transdermal	Fentanyl (patches)	It is abused by scraping the contents and smoking them

In many areas of Mexico, tramadol is mixed with soda, marijuana, or alcohol, and sold without a prescription.

4.6.2.2 Mechanism of action: Trick Pain, Trick the Brain

Opioids mimic endorphins, the body's natural pain-relieving substances. They bind to μ-opioid receptors and produce:

- Profound analgesia.
- Emotional euphoria.
- Physical sedation.
- Respiratory depression.

But repeated use reduces the natural production of endorphins, and the body enters a state of biochemical dependence (Figure 13).

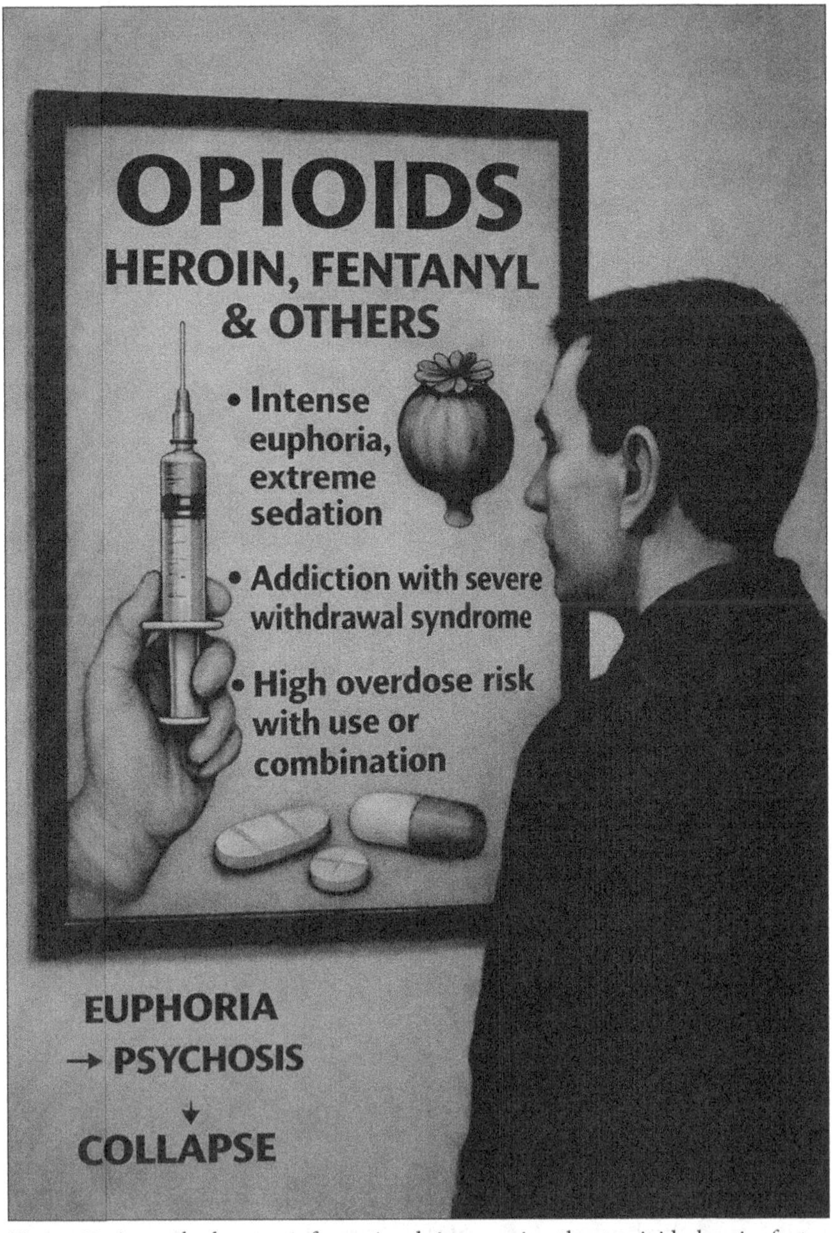

Figure 13. A man looks at an informational sign warning about opioids: heroin, fentanyl and others. The image highlights the dangers of intense euphoria, extreme sedation, strong withdrawal syndrome, and high risk of overdose. A silent scene that reflects the moment of awareness before a critical decision.

4.6.3 Heroin: the Drug that "Embraces" and Abandons

It is derived from morphine, but 2–3 times more potent. On the street it is known as "la H", "caballo", "blanca", "choco" and "blacktar". When injected, the "rush" is immediate: a sensation that addicts describe as "orgasm multiplied by a thousand": "You feel like you're floating in warm water... and then everything else stops mattering".

In Mexico and the United States, heroin is increasingly mixed with fentanyl, without the user's knowledge.

4.6.4 Fentanyl: the Molecule of Silence

- Lethal dose: 2 mg (size of 3 grains of salt).
- On the street he is known as "devil", "ghost", "Chinese dust", and "the 50".

   1- Very lipophilic → crosses the brain in seconds.

   2- Causes respiratory arrest without warning; Many users die in their sleep, with the syringe still in their veins.

In cities like San Francisco or Ciudad Juárez, morgues report weekly spikes in fentanyl deaths in teens.

How does the "hook" occur?

- First exposure (physical pain, surgery, accident).
- Feeling of relief + euphoria.
- Repetition → neuroadaptation.
- Increased tolerance → higher doses.
- Withdrawal syndrome → consumption to avoid suffering.
- Desperation → mixing with alcohol, benzodiazepines, or stimulants.

End: overdose, hospitalization, or death (Figure 14).

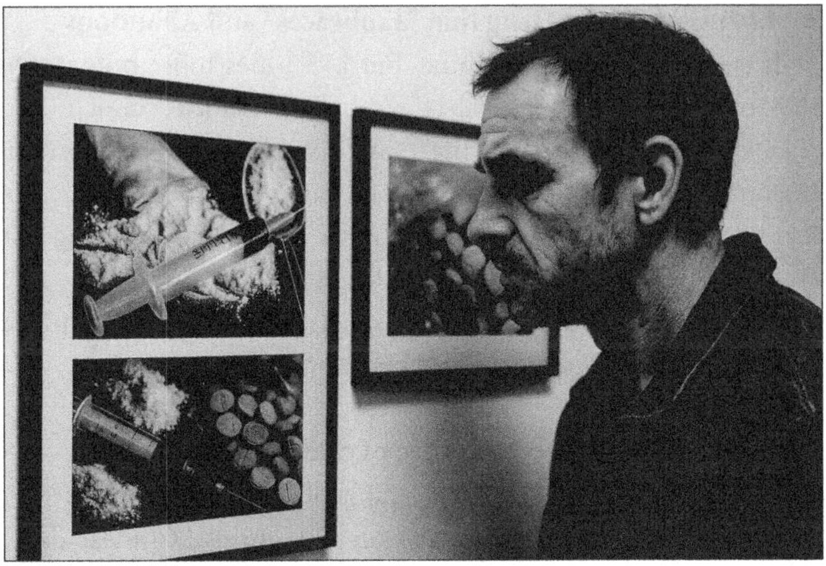

Figure 14. A man looks anxiously at photographs of synthetic drugs and colorful pills, representing the growing risk of new designer drugs, whose harmless appearance hides a high potential for addiction, overdose and severe neurological disorders.

Abstinence: Skinless Hell

Phase	Physical symptoms	Emotional Symptoms
6-24h	Bone pain, tremors, vomiting, diarrhea	Anxiety, panic, anger, insomnia
Day 2-5	Heavy sweating, fever, goosebumps	Deep depression, hopelessness
Day 6-10	Extreme fatigue, overflowing appetite	Intense craving , suicidal impulsivity

Clinical Testimony

"I felt like my flesh was being ripped off, but inside" (30-year-old man in heroin withdrawal).

Clinical Treatment: from Rescue to Rehabilitation

Emergency: overdose

- Naloxone (Narcan): Opioid antagonist, life-saving if given in time.
- Nasal or intramuscular.
- Available over the counter in the United States, scarce in Mexico and Spain.

In many community centers, people are already trained to carry naloxone as if it were a first aid kit.

Long-term Treatment

Drug	Clinical Advantages
Methadone	Stabilizes the patient, prevents craving
Buprenorphine	Lower risk of overdose, ceiling effect
Naltrexona	Completely blocks euphoric effects
Psychiatric accompaniment	Management of depression, anxiety, PTSD

Psychotherapy:

- Cognitive behavioral therapy (relapse prevention).
- 12-step groups (NA).
- Psychodynamic psychotherapy (childhood trauma, grief).

Clinical cases

Clinical case 1. "It Wasn't Physical Pain"

Carla, 29 years old, survivor of child abuse. He used prescription tramadol at 17. At 22 he was already using heroin IV. She was found unconscious in a public restroom. 12-month rehabilitation with methadone and trauma therapy.

Clinical case 2. "A Simple Patch"

Gerardo, 52 years old, nurse with low back pain. He stole fentanyl patches from the hospital. By scraping and inhaling them, he had 3 overdoses in a month. Today he lives in a rural community with religious and psychological accompaniment.

4.7 Benzodiazepines, Anxiolytics and Lethal Combinations

4.7.1 The Relief Trap: How Sleep Becomes Dependency

Benzodiazepines (BZDs) were hailed in the 1960s as the pharmacological miracle against anxiety, insomnia, and panic attacks. But over time, these same molecules became one of the most common causes of inadvertent dependence, accidental overdoses, and cognitive decline.

Nowadays millions of people consume them without knowing that they can generate addiction similar to opioids, especially when combined with these, alcohol or barbiturates.

4.7.2 Main Benzodiazepines and Anxiolytics

Substance	Trade Name (Best Known)	Half-life	Clinical Comments
Alprazolam	Xanax	Short (6-12 h)	High potency, fast effect → increased addiction
Clonazepam	Rivotril	Intermedia (18-50 h)	Chronic anxiety, epilepsy
Lorazepam	Ativan	Intermedia (10-20 h)	Useful in psychiatric emergencies

Substance	Trade Name (Best Known)	Half-life	Clinical Comments
Diazepam	Valium	Long (20-100 h)	Used in Alcoholic Detoxification
Triazolam	Halcion	Very short (2-6 h)	Severe insomnia; High risk of amnesia
Midazolam	Dormicum	Ultracta (1-4 h)	Hospital/Anesthesia Use

There are also non-BZD anxiolytics such as zolpidem, zopiclone or buspirone, with lower risk but similar effects.

4.7.3 Action Mechanism: the Switch of the GABA System

BZDs work by boosting GABA, the brain's main inhibitory neurotransmitter. This causes:

- Sedation.
- Decreased anxiety.
- Muscle relaxation.
- Reduced epileptic activity.

But prolonged use reduces the sensitivity of the GABA-A receptor, leading to tolerance, dependence, and withdrawal.

4.7.4 Desired Effects and Correct Clinical Use

Legitimate Medical Indication	Suggested Duration	Risks if Prolonged
Acute insomnia	Maximum 2 weeks	Dependence, insomnia, rebound
Generalized anxiety disorders	≤ 4–6 weeks	Cognitive decline, emotional dysfunction
Panic attacks	Spot use (rescue)	Psychological addiction
Seizure or catatonia	Clinical Emergencies	Brief hospital use

Clinical Testimony

"My psychiatrist gave me alprazolam for anxiety. Six years later I can't sleep without it. They prescribe it to me as if they were candy" (34-year-old woman).

4.7.5 Side Effects and Harms from Chronic Use

Cognitive Effects:

- Anterograde amnesia.
- Attention and concentration deficit.
- Depersonalization.
- Psychomotor slowdown.
- Increased risk of dementia in the long term.

Emotional Effects:

- Affective flattening.
- Emotional lability.
- Secondary depression.

Recent studies link long-term use of BZDs to hippocampal atrophy and reduced neuroplasticity (Figure 15).

4.7.6 Lethal Combinations: Fatal Synergies

Combination	Clinical Outcome
BZD + alcohol	Respiratory depression, coma, death
BZD+ opioids (heroin, fentanyl)	Lethal synergy → respiratory arrest
BZD + Barbiturates	Extreme risk of amnesia, coma
BZD+ stimulants (cocaine, methamphetamine)	Impaired judgment → impulsivity, suicide

More than 70% of fentanyl overdoses include benzodiazepines in toxicological autopsy.

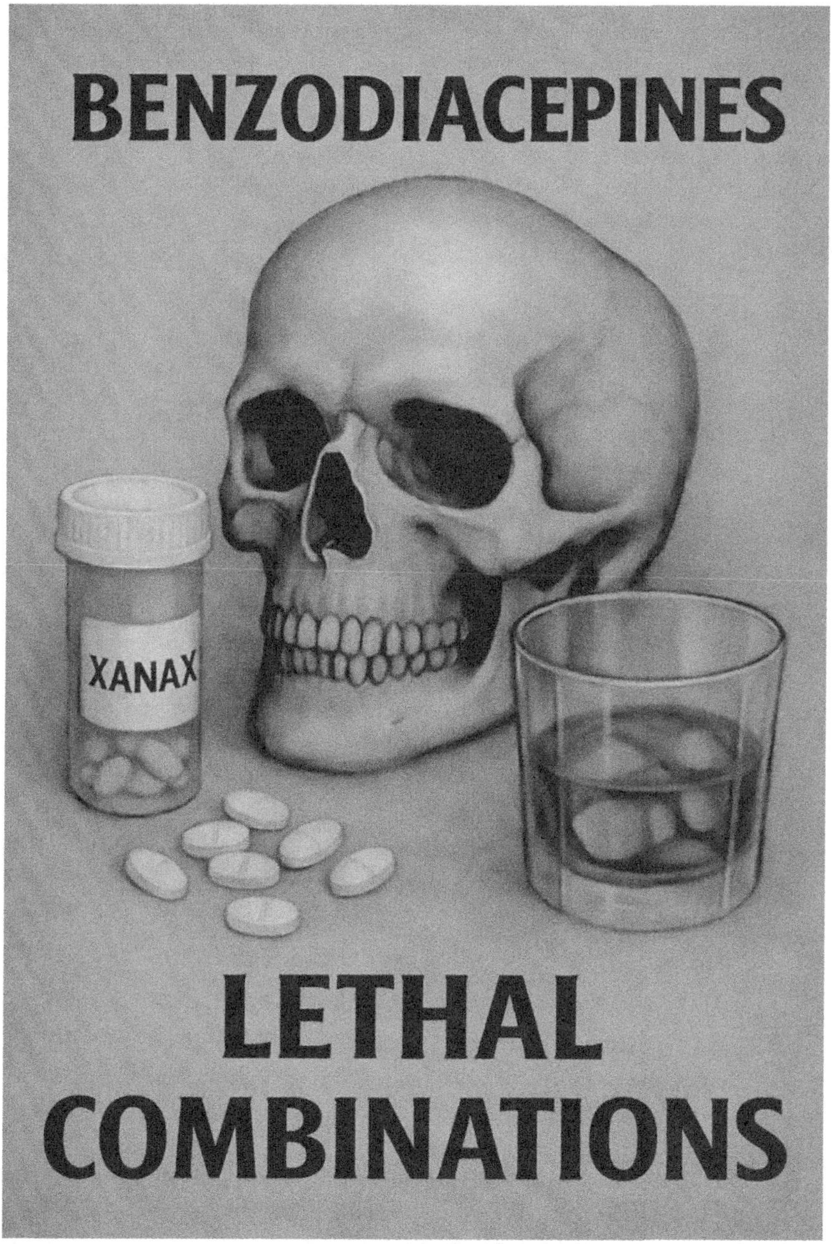

Figure 15. A skull accompanies a bottle of benzodiazepines and a glass of alcohol, representing the mortal risk of combinations between anxiolytics and central nervous system depressants. What seems like a relief can turn into a fatal sentence.

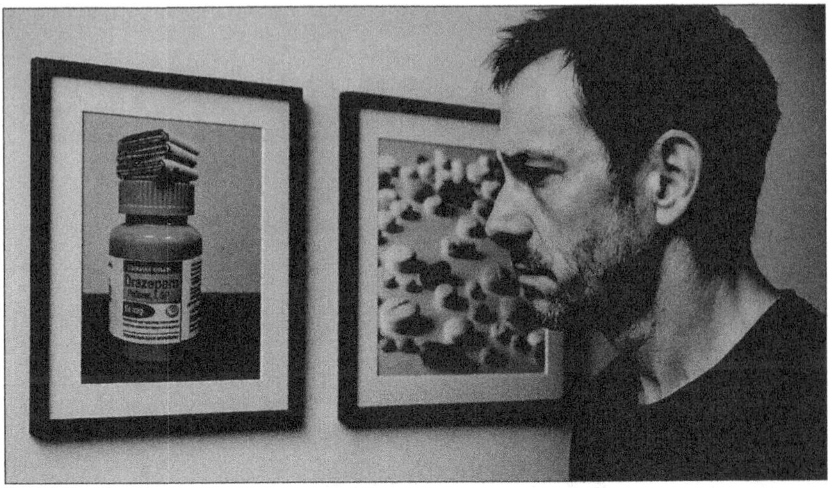

Figure 16. A man stares with concern at photographs of anti-anxiety drugs and prescription pills, symbolizing the silent dependence that many people develop when seeking relief from sleep or calming anxiety. What starts as treatment can become a chemical trap.

4.7.7 Benzodiazepine Withdrawal: a Brain Storm

Symptoms:

- Insomnius severus.
- Intense anxiety, panic.
- Hypersensitivity to light, sound, and touch.
- Tremors, seizures.
- Obsessive ideas, depression, suicidal ideation.
- Derealization and depersonalization syndrome.

Abrupt withdrawal can cause seizures and death, especially after prolonged use.

4.7.8 Treatment of Benzodiazepine Dependence

Main strategy: tapering (supervised tapering)

- Weekly dose reduction: 5-10%.
- Transition to a BZD with a long half-life (example: diazepam).
- Ongoing psychological support (Figure 16).

4.7.9 Adjuvant medication

Drug	Therapeutic Function
SSRI antidepressants	Anxiety control during the process
Anticonvulsants (gabapentin)	Reduction of somatic symptoms
Trazodone, mirtazapine	Sleep without generating new addiction
Melatonin	Circadian rhythm restructuring

Clinical cases

Clinical case 1. Inadvertent Addiction

Daniel, 44 years old. He had been using alprazolam for 8 years. When he tried to quit abruptly, he developed seizures. She required hospitalization and slow withdrawal with diazepam. Today he has been free for 15 months on CBT therapy.

Clinical case 2. Combined Overdose

Rocío, 25, smoked fentanyl and took clonazepam. He suffered a respiratory arrest. Revived with naloxone on the street. Currently in a therapeutic community with benzodiazepine reduction and buprenorphine use.

4.8 Inhalants: Active, "Mona", Gasoline, Tiner

4.8.1 The Silent Poison: Toxic, Street and Childhood Addiction

Inhalants are volatile chemicals that produce psychoactive effects when inhaled. They are cheap, accessible and legal in many regions, making them **one of the first drugs used among children and adolescents living on the streets** (Figure 17).

In Latin America, the use of "mona" or "active" is endemic among minors living in extreme poverty or family abandonment.

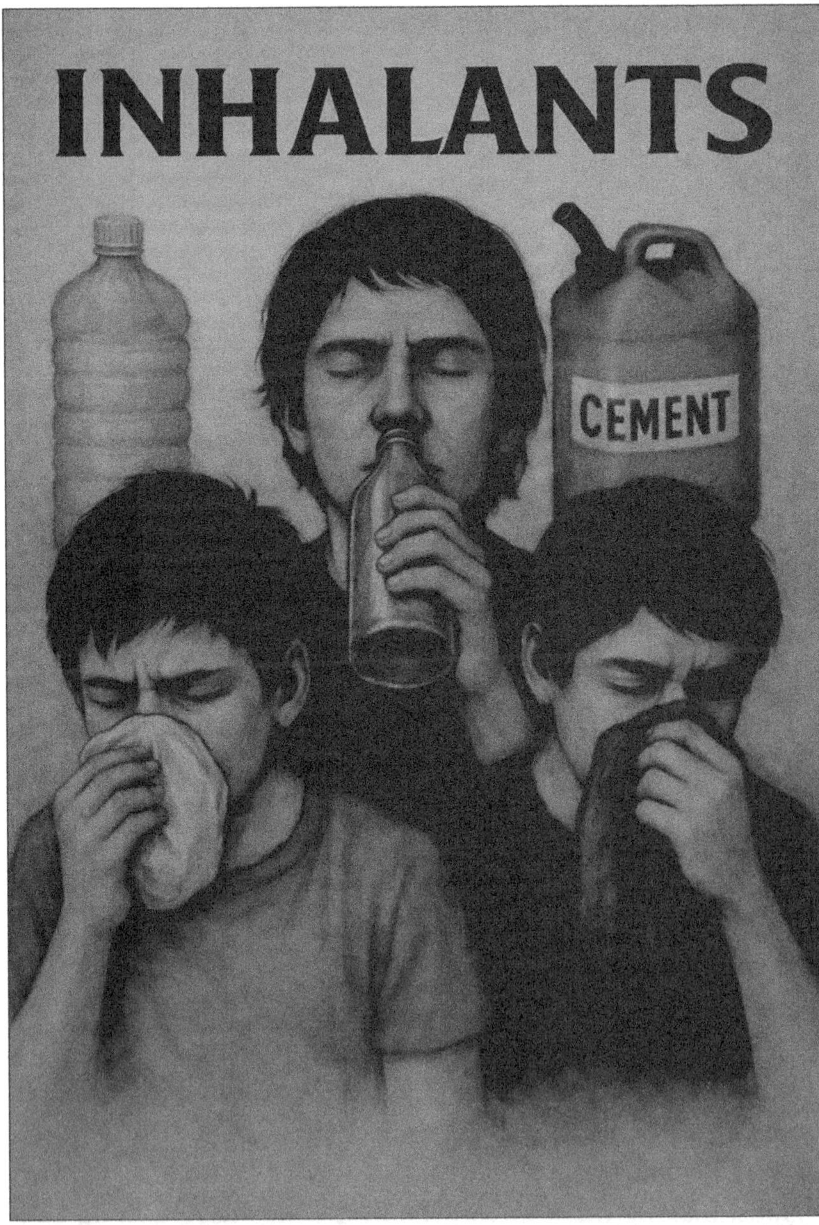

Figure 17. Three children inhale substances from bottles and rags, surrounded by cement containers and solvents. The image represents one of the most invisible and devastating forms of childhood addiction, marked by poverty, abandonment and irreversible neurological damage.

4.8.2 Substances Used and Street Names

Substance	Street Name	Original Use	How to Use
Toluene	"Mona", "active", tinker	Industrial solvent	Inhaled into bags or rags
Gasoline	Gas, 93, diesel	Fuel	Direct smell, bag, rag
Ether	Flown, Aether	Anesthesia, solvent	Continuous inhalation
Pegamento (Pega)	Cemento, the crazy one	Industrial adhesive	Inhaled by nose or mouth
Nitrates (poppers)	Rush, aroma, poppers	Sexual vasodilator	Inhaled at parties (Figure 18)

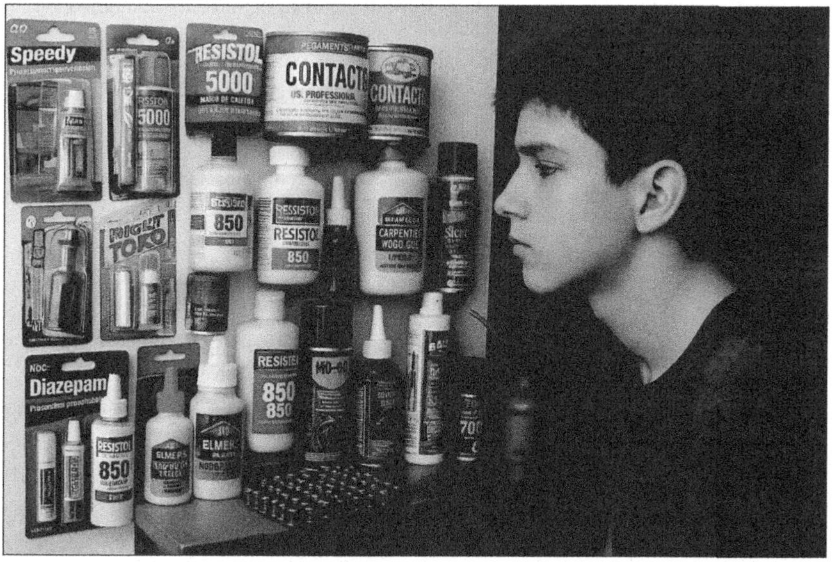

Figure 18. A teenager stares at a collection of industrial solvents, glues, oils and toxic products, many of which are used as inhalants in street consumption contexts. The scene depicts the everyday and dangerous access to these legal substances, and the fine line between domestic use and addictive abuse.

In Mexico, the term "andarse con la mona" is used to describe the young man who walks around drugged with a bag on his face.

4.8.3 Mechanism of Action: Central Nervous System Anesthesia

Inhalants depress the CNS by:

- Dissolution of neuronal lipids.
- Inhibition of NMDA receptors.
- Transient increase in dopamine and brief euphoria.

Most of its components are **neurotoxic**, **hepatotoxic** and **cardiotoxic**, even with few exposures.

4.8.4 Immediate Effects of Consumption

Minutes after Inhalation	Acute Effects
0–2 minutes	Euphoria, dizziness, uncontrollable laughter
2–5 minutes	Disinhibition, alteration of judgment
5–10 minutes	Drowsiness, blurred vision, unsteadiness
10–30 minutes	Hallucinations, aggression, nausea
>30 minutes	Unconsciousness, arrhythmias, sudden death

Repeated use in the same session is known as "chain sniffing".

4.8.5 Chronic damage: every Inhalation, a Slow Death

Neurological:

- Brain atrophy visible on neuroimaging.
- Dementia praecox, cerebellar syndrome (unstable gait).

- Peripheral polyneuropathy.
- Seizures, paralysis.

Psychiatric:
- Inhalant psychosis.
- Irritability, impulsivity, behavioral disorders.
- Affective flattening, acquired autism.

Other bodies:
- Chemical hepatitis.
- Toxic nephritis.
- Cardiomyopathy.
- Leukopenia, immunosuppression.

The heart can **stop suddenly** in the face of a rush of adrenaline → **sudden inhalation death syndrome**.

4.8.6 Social and Demographic Context

- 70% of consumers are **under the age of 18**.
- 90% live on **the streets, orphans or abandoned**.
- Inhalants are used to "**kill hunger, fear, or cold**".
- Many consumers start before the age of **10**.
- Most affected areas: Mexico, Central America, Brazil, India and the Philippines.

Clinical Testimony

"When I have a monkey I no longer remember that I am hungry" (12-year-old boy in Mexico City).

Treatment Difficulties:
- Extreme stigmatization.
- Lack of motivation due to cognitive impairment.
- Abandonment of treatment due to mental disorganization.
- High recidivism.

Effective strategies:

- Extended residential rehabilitation.
- Structured occupational therapy.
- Family and community support.
- Group psychotherapy based on routine and safety.
- Street interventions with intensive follow-up.

Clinical cases

Clinical case 1. Child Chronic Inhaler

Andrés, 11 years old. He lives under a bridge. Inhale active from the age of 7. He does not know how to read or write. He has an unsteady gait and difficulty speaking. Rescued by civil foundation. Diagnosis: Toluene dementia, cerebellar syndrome, and severe malnutrition.

Clinical case 2. Institutionalized Adolescent

Luz, 15 years old. Kicked out of her home for sexual abuse. Consume ether in public restrooms. She was admitted with chemical hepatitis. Under the tutelage of the DIF. Positive evolution after 8 months of hospitalization and therapeutic school.

4.9 Hallucinogens and Psychedelic Drugs

4.9.1 Doors of Perception, Abysses of Mind

Hallucinogens and psychedelics have accompanied humans since prehistoric times: in shamanic rituals, mystical visions, and philosophical explorations. However, outside of controlled contexts, its consumption can trigger psychiatric crises, psychological dependence, and persistent traumas (Figure 19).

Today they resurface under a new mask: psychedelic therapies for depression and post-traumatic stress. But its recreational use remains a dangerous and poorly understood reality.

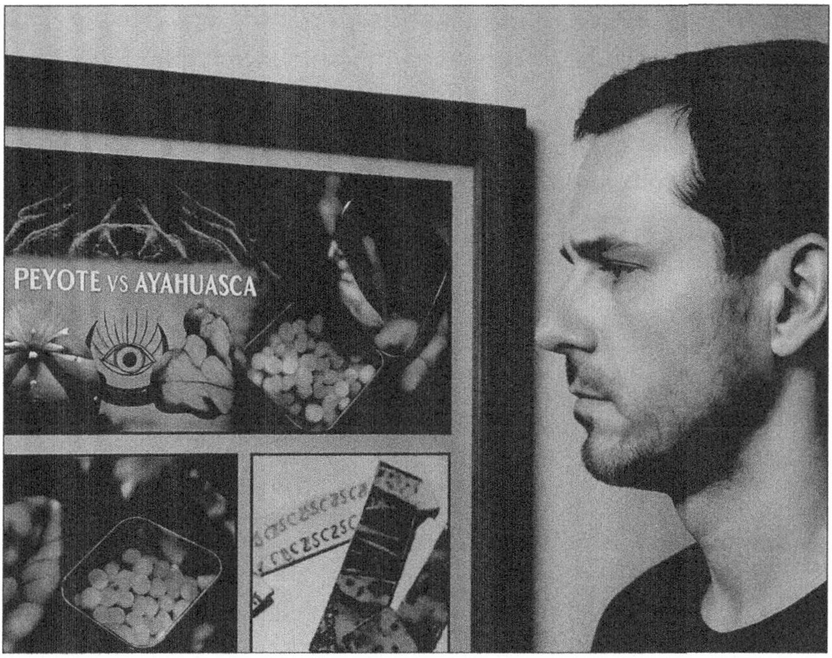

Figure 19. A man contemplates a chart comparing different hallucinogenic and psychedelic substances such as peyote, ayahuasca, LSD and synthetic pills. The scene represents the threshold between the spiritual quest, the expansion of consciousness, and the psychological risks of these visionary compounds.

4.9.2 Classification of Hallucinogens and Psychedelics

Type	Common Substances	Main Effect
Tryptamines.	LSD, psilocybin (magic mushrooms), DMT	Perceptual distortion, synesthesia, spiritual vision
Phenethylamines	Mescalina, MDMA, 2C-B	Emotional, visual and tactile stimulation
Anticholinergics	Datura, scopolamine	Delirium, amnesia, frightening hallucinations
Dissociatives	Ketamine, PCP, DXM	Depersonalization, separation of body and mind

Many substances appear as “drops”, “powders”, “papers”, or “gummies”. In Cuba, synthetic compounds such as NBOMe are called “the chemist” or “the little paper”.

4.9.3 Mechanism of action: opening the doors of consciousness too wide

- Psychedelics act as agonists of 5-HT2A (serotonin) receptors, altering perception, time, self, and the environment.
- Being dissociative, they block NMDA receptors, creating out-of-body experiences.

Over-activation of these pathways can trigger psychosis in vulnerable people, even with a single dose.

4.9.4 Immediate Effects of Consumption

Start Time	Possible Effects
20-60 min	Visual distortion, bright colors, euphoria.
1-3 hours	Hallucinations, synesthesia, existential revelations.
4-6 hours	Confusion, paranoia, panic.
6-12 hours	Fatigue, mental exhaustion, “difficult journey”.
Days or weeks	Flashbacks, HPPD (persistent perceptual disorder).

Clinical Testimony

“I felt like I was floating out of my body, then I heard voices for weeks” (LSD user, 23 years old).

4.9.5 Psychiatric and Physical Risks

Psychological:

- Induced psychosis (schizophrenia type).

- Anxiety disorders or prolonged panic.
- Unintentional flashbacks.
- HPPD (permanent visual hallucinations).
- Dissociative syndrome.

Physical:

- Increased blood pressure and temperature.
- Seizures (especially with NBOMe or adulterated LSD).
- High-risk behaviors (accidents, suicide).

There are reports of patients who tried to **fly out of the window** during a "trip", or threw themselves into the sea "to merge with the universo".

4.9.6 Contexts of consumption: Spirituality, Celebration, Self-exploration

- Traditional rituals: ayahuasca, peyote, mushrooms, bufotenin.
- Electronic parties: LSD, MDMA, ketamine, 2C-B.
- Self-medication: microdosing for depression or anxiety.
- Marginal urban context: NBOMe, DXM of cough syrups (Figure 20).

Microdoses (LSD or psilocybin in subperceptual doses) are being studied, but there is still no solid clinical evidence of long-term efficacy or safety.

Clinical cases

Clinical case 1. Mystical Crisis with Psychotic Relapse

Martín, 34 years old. He took ayahuasca at a retreat. He experienced "spiritual rebirth", but two weeks later he began to hear voices and believed he was chosen by the universe. Diagnosed with acute psychotic episode. Hospitalized for 30 days.

Clinical case 2. Teen in Rave

Julia, 17 years old. He took 2C-B at electronic party. He assaulted a colleague, believing that he was "an evil shadow". She was admitted with psychotic agitation. Treated with antipsychotics. He dropped out of school due to cognitive sequelae.

4.9.7 Treatment of Complications

- **Benzodiazepines:** for acute anxiety or bad travel.
- **Atypical antipsychotics:** if there is persistent psychosis.
- **Cognitive-behavioral therapy:** integration of experience and prevention of relapse.
- **Family psychoeducation:** key in young people with first outbreaks.
- **Physical containment + safe environment:** essential in emergencies.

4.10 New Designer Drugs and Emerging Substances

4.10.1 The Chaos Lab: the Addiction that Still Has no Name

New designer drugs (NPS) are psychoactive substances created to simulate the effects of illegal drugs (such as cannabis, cocaine, LSD, or MDMA), but with modified chemical structures that bypass legal control. They appear and disappear quickly in the clandestine market, making them difficult to detect, regulate and treat (Figure 21).

More than **1,000 NPS have been documented since 2009**. Many of them are **more potent**, **more toxic**, and **more unpredictable** than traditional drugs.

4.10.2 General Classification of NPS

Major Group	Known Examples	Simulated Effects
Synthetic cannabinoids	K2, Spice, Black Mamba, Joker	Cannabis, but with a higher risk of psychosis
Synthetic cathinones	Flakka, MDPV, "bath salts"	Stimulants such as cocaine or methamphetamine

Major Group	Known Examples	Simulated Effects
Synthetic opioids	U-47700, W-18, isotonitazeno	Heroin or fentanyl, much more potent
Phenylethylamines	2C-B, 2C-I, NBOMe	LSD, MDMA, mescalina
Synthetic benzodiazepines	Etizolam, flualprazolam	Anxiolytics, hypnotics
New Dissociatives	MXE, 3-MeO-PCP, ketamina "china"	Ketamina, PCP

Why are they so dangerous?

- **Unknown potency** → easily overdosed.
- **Variable composition** → each batch may be different.
- **No specific antidotes.**
- **Difficult to detect in toxicological tests.**
- **High possibility of psychosis, seizures, sudden death.**

A single Spice cigarette can cause **catatonia**, **agitated delirium**, or **cardiorespiratory arrest** (Figure 22).

4.10.3 Observed Clinical Effects

Affected System	Typical Manifestations
Neurological	Seizures, psychosis, coma, severe paranoia
Cardiac	Tachycardia, hypertension, heart attack
Psychiatric	Extreme agitation, suicide attempt, aggression
Hepatic and renal	Acute hepatitis, acute kidney failure
Behavioral	Depersonalization, mystical or paranoid delusions

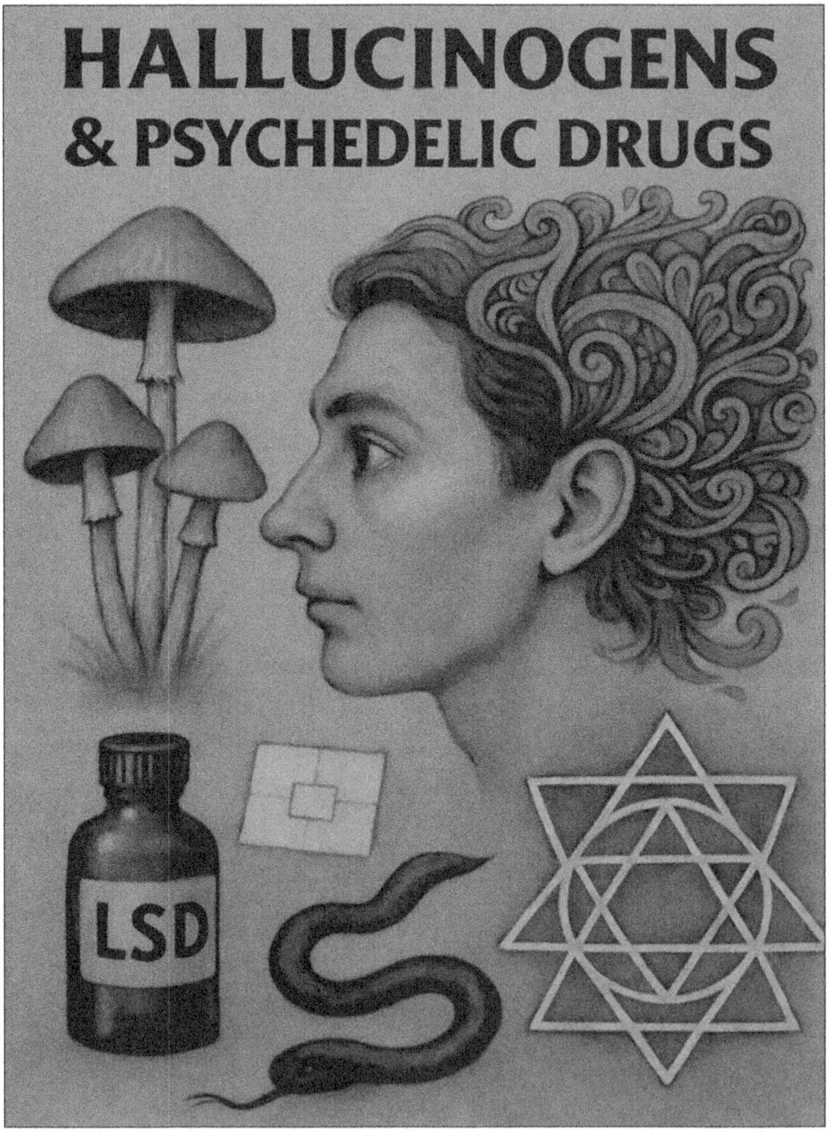

Figure 20. Symbolic representation of the use of hallucinogens and psychedelic drugs: mushrooms, LSD and mystical symbols allude to experiences of expansion of consciousness, deep introspection and spiritual contact, but also to the risks of psychic disintegration.

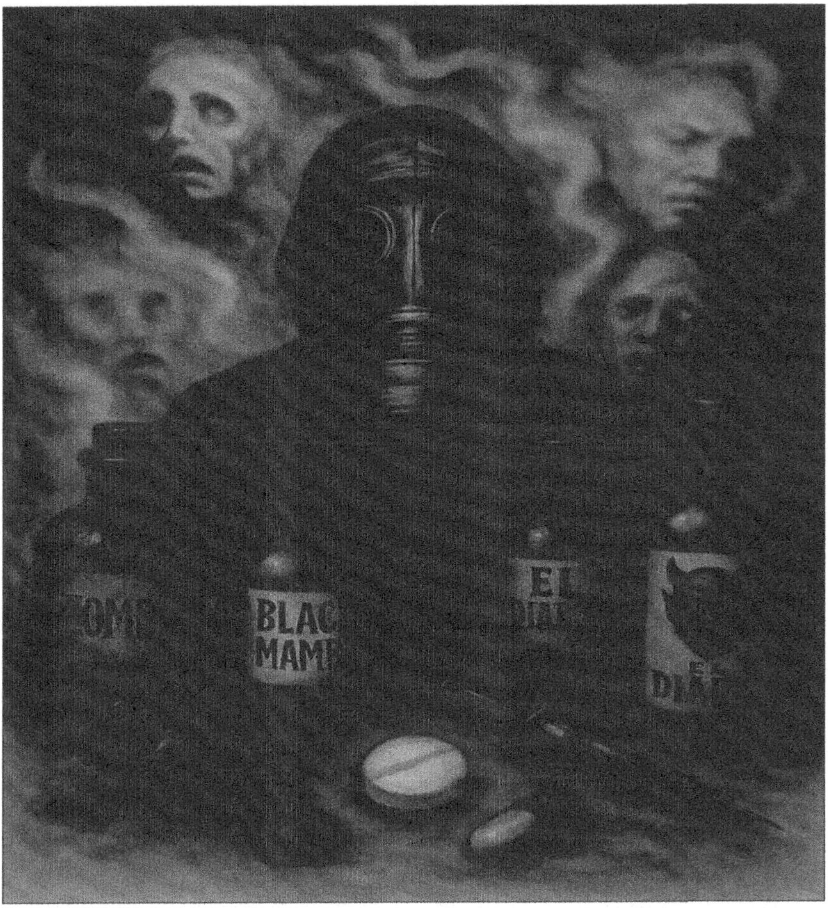

Figure 21. A hooded man with a gas mask represents the mystery and danger of new designer drugs. Labels such as "zombie", "black mamba" and "the devil" evoke the extreme, unknown and terrifying effects of these substances, often created in clandestine laboratories without regulation or antidote.

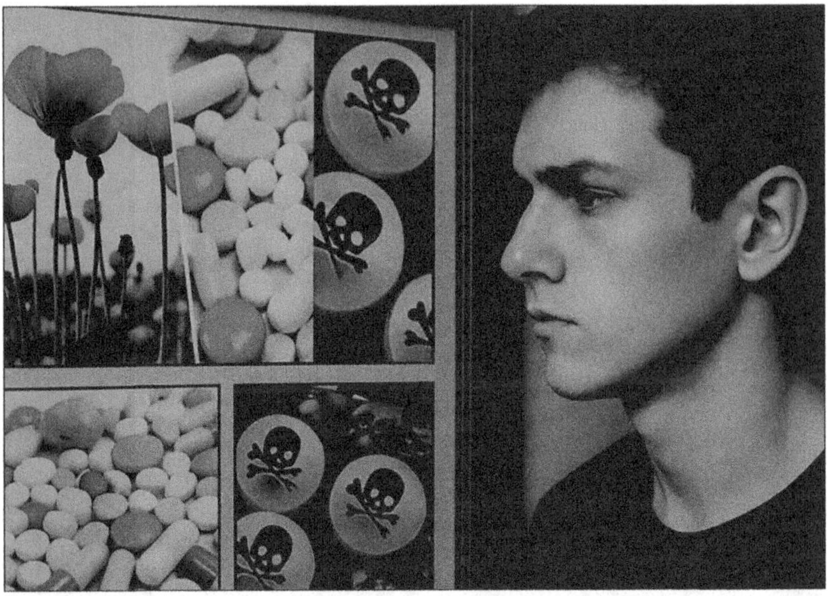

Figure 22. A young man looks at a gallery of colorful, seemingly harmless pills marked with danger symbols. This image denounces the growing threat of new designer drugs, many disguised as candy or medicines, whose true effect can be lethal and devastating to the brain.

4.10.4 Consumption Modes

- Smoked (mixed with tobacco or marijuana).
- Inhaled (powders or "crystals").
- In drops (NBOMe, liquid cannabinoids).
- In "ecstasy" tablets or capsules.
- Injected (some cathinones or opioids).

Many times users **do not know what they are consuming**. For example, they think they smoke marijuana, but it's a synthetic cannabinoid sprayed.

Clinical cases

Clinical case 1. Spice seizures

Marcos, 18 years old. He smoked what he believed was "gas station marijuana". Within minutes he had seizures, foaming at the mouth and muscle stiffness. Diagnosis: synthetic cannabinoid poisoning. Hospitalization in ICU, partial recovery with mild cognitive impairment.

Clinical case 2. Psychotic Break with NBOMe

Angela, 21 years old. He took a piece of paper at a party. Hours later she thought she was being chased by demons, she injured herself with a knife. Prolonged psychiatric hospitalization. Diagnosis: Unknown substance-induced psychosis, suspicion of NBOMe.

4.10.5 Clinical Approach and Medical Challenges

- There is no specific treatment in most cases.
- Symptomatic management is used: benzodiazepines, antipsychotics, hydration.
- Need for ICU in overdose with synthetic opioids.
- Absence of markers in standard exams.
- Instability of the condition → can change from sedation to aggression in minutes.

4.10.6 Prevention and Surveillance

- International monitoring: UN, EMCDDA, DEA.
- Real-time alert applications.
- Community education: **if you don't know what's in it, don't use it.**
- Training of medical and paramedical personnel in clinical identification.

4.11 Combination Drugs and Polydrug Use Syndrome

4.11.1 When the Body Becomes a Lethal Laboratory

Polydrug use is the practice of using two or more drugs at the same time or in continuous sequence. It can be intentional (to enhance or soften effects) or accidental (due to ignorance of the content of street substances). It is common in chronic users, in party or street contexts, and exponentially increases toxicity, unpredictability and the risk of death (Figure 23).

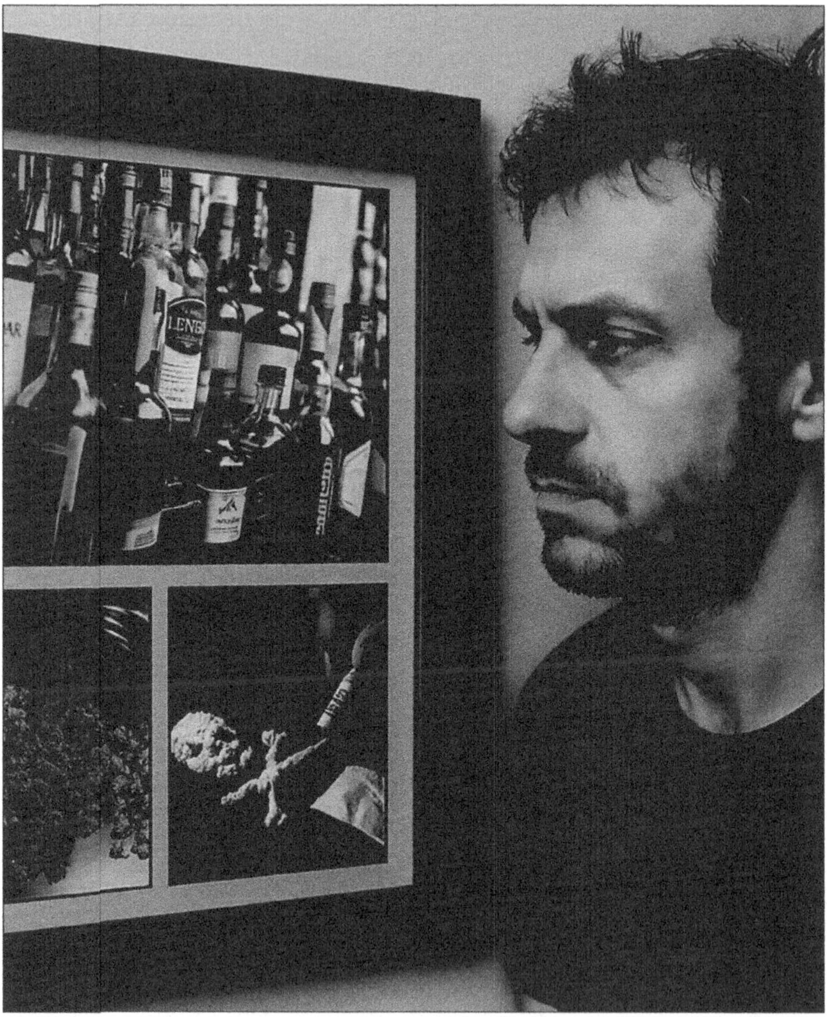

Figure 23. A man contemplates, with a worried expression, a visual composition showing alcohol, marijuana and cocaine, which symbolizes polydrug use syndrome. The mixture of substances turns the human body into a chaotic laboratory, where each combination can trigger unpredictable and deadly reactions.

Today, more than 65% of fatal overdoses in America involve multiple substances.

4.11.2 Common Types of Combinations

Usual Combination	Street Name/ Culture	Target
Alcohol + cocaine	"Latin Speedball"	Enhance euphoria + reduce anxiety.
Heroin + cocaine	Classic "Speedball"	Going up and down at the same time (maximum risk).
Benzodiazepines + opioids	"Cocktail of death"	Increasing sedation, "turning off the world".
MDMA + LSD	"Candyflip"	Merging emotional stimulus and psychedelia.
Marijuana + alcohol	"Crossfaded"	Intensification of distortion and drowsiness
Tramadol + clonaze-pam	"Tachas 225" (in Mexico)	Cheap, easy to get, highly addictive

Many people don't know that **ecstasy or marijuana can be adulterated with fentanyl, methamphetamine, or NBOMe**.

4.11.3 Pathophysiology of Polydrug Use

The human body is not designed to process multiple psychoactive substances simultaneously. The combined effect can be:

- **Synergistic** (1 + 1 = 3): as opioids + benzos → greater respiratory depression.

- **Antagonistic** (1 – 1 = confusion): such as cocaine + heroin → opposite effects that overload the cardiovascular system.

- **Multiplier** (1 x 1 = 10): LSD + MDMA + cannabis → total dissociation, psychotic breakdown.

The liver, kidneys, and nervous system collapse under unpredictable toxic interactions.

4.11.4 Clinical Manifestations of Polydrug Use

Affected System	Characteristic Symptoms
Brain	Seizures, coma, acute psychosis, delirium
Heart	Arrhythmias, acute infarction, hemodynamic collapse
Breathing	Bradypnea, apnea, respiratory arrest
Psychism	Depersonalization, severe anxiety, panic attacks
Conduct	Extreme agitation, violence, self-harm, suicide

4.11.5 The Special Case of the Speedball

One of the **deadliest combinations** in the history of drug addiction:

- Heroin (depressant) + Cocaine (stimulant).
- Feeling of "false balance" → the user does not perceive an imminent overdose.
- Cocaine acts fast and goes fast.
- Heroin remains longer → **respiratory arrest after the "crash"**.

Famous speedball deaths: **John Belushi, River Phoenix, Philip Seymour Hoffman**.

4.11.6 Combinations in Current Contexts

- **Electronic parties:** MDMA + ketamine + LSD + alcohol → panic attacks, collapse, dehydration.
- **Streets of Latin America:** active + clonazepam + tramadol + marijuana → cognitive impairment, psychotic breaks.

- **Universities:** Adderall + alcohol + marijuana → emotional overload, induced psychosis.

- **Clandestine hospitals:** patients hospitalized with 3-5 substances in their blood without knowing it.

Clinical cases

Clinical case 1. Combined Overdose at Rave

Lucas, 24 years old. He took LSD, MDMA and alcohol at a festival. He ended up stripping naked, screaming "I am God" and convulsed on the ground. Taken to the emergency room, he had to be intubated. Diagnosis: acute toxic encephalopathy due to polydrug use.

Clinical case 2. Teenager in a Street Situation

Emilia, 15 years old. He inhaled "mona", took studs (tramadol + clonazepam) and smoked marijuana mixed with crystal. He was admitted with paranoid delirium and signs of extreme malnutrition. Diagnosis: multiple withdrawal syndrome + induced psychosis.

4.11.7 Treatment of Polydrug Use

- **Multiple toxicological evaluation** (if possible).
- **Symptomatic management:** benzodiazepines, antipsychotics, fluid therapy.
- **Controlled and quiet environment.**
- **Continuous monitoring** in the ICU if there is respiratory depression or seizure.
- **Gradual and phased detoxification** (prioritizing the most dangerous).
- **Intensive psychotherapy** and community follow-up.

Treatment must be tailored on a case-by-case basis, as each mixture is unique.

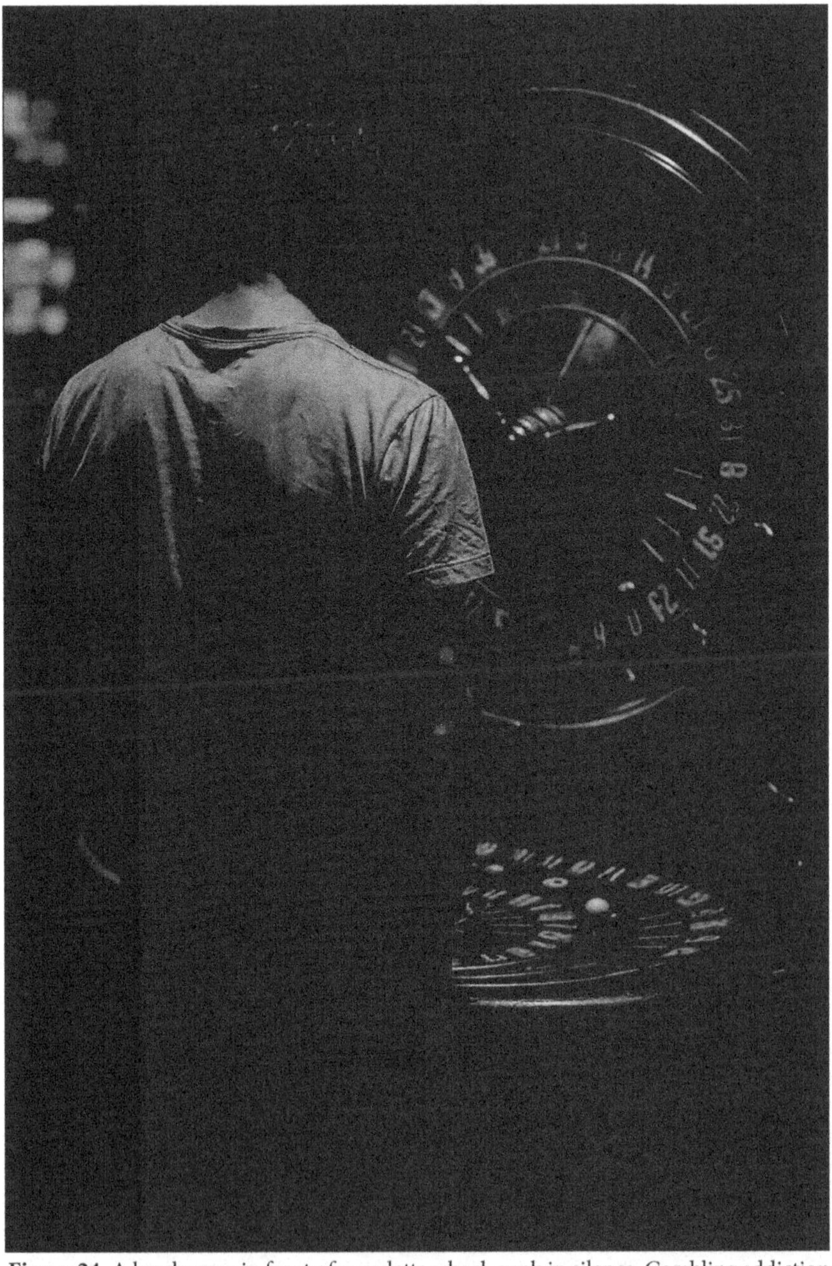

Figure 24. A lonely man in front of a roulette wheel, sunk in silence. Gambling addiction transforms hope into obsession, trapping the brain in a cycle of illusion, loss, and guilt.

CHAPTER 5
Addictions without Substance. When the Compulsion is Lodged in the Behavior

5.1 Gambling Addiction (Compulsive Gambling)

5.1.1 When Chance Becomes Prison: the Brain Trapped in the Promise of Winning

There is no smoke, no syringe, no drink. There is no smell of drugs or obvious physical deterioration. But there is ruin. There is anxiety, despair, lies, debt, loneliness, and, in many cases, suicide. Gambling addiction is one of the most invisible—and devastating—forms of addiction. The pathological gambler does not seek pleasure: he seeks relief from emptiness. He does not play to win: he plays not to feel.

5.1.2 What is Gambling Addiction?

Pathological gambling disorder is a behavioural addiction characterised by the loss of control over gambling behaviour, despite its negative personal, family, work and legal consequences. It is recognized in the DSM-5 and ICD-11 as an impulse control disorder, with criteria similar to substance addictions (Figure 24).

5.1.3 Neurobiology of the Compulsive Gambler

- Dopamine: every time you play, the reward circuit is activated. The expectation of winning—even if you lose—produces a dopamine rush in the nucleus accumbens.

- Mesolimbic system: the same one that is activated with cocaine, heroin or sex, responds here to the "near-win" or near-miss, which reinforces the behavior.

- Cognitive distortions: such as the "illusion of control", "player bias" or "magical thinking", where the subject believes that chance can influence them.

- Tolerance and abstinence: the player needs to bet more and more money, more often and, if he does not, he experiences anxiety, irritability and insomnia.

5.1.4 Summary Diagnostic Criteria (DSM-5)

- Constant preoccupation with gambling.
- Need to bet increasing sums.
- Repeated failure to quit.
- Lies, loss of relationships, theft.
- Use play as an escape route.
- Relapses after quitting.
- Efforts to recover lost money (the "double or nothing" trap).

It is diagnosed if there are at least 4 criteria in the last 12 months, and is classified as mild, moderate or severe.

5.1.5 Profile of the Pathological Gambler

- Age: it can begin in adolescence or old age.
- Sex: more frequent in men, although in women it is usually more progressive and associated with loneliness.
- Entry route: sports betting, slot machines, lottery, online casinos, mobile games.
- Comorbidities: ADHD, depression, bipolar disorder, borderline disorder, substance use, anxiety.

5.1.6 What Triggers it?

- Individual factors: impulsivity, sensation seeking, low self-esteem.
- Family history of gambling or addiction.
- Social environment: promotion of gambling as innocent entertainment or as an escape.

- Technology: online gaming, app betting, 24/7 targeted advertising.
- Life events: bereavement, unemployment, separation, illness.

5.1.7 A Disease without Substance, but with the Same Chains

Gambling addiction is a "dry" addiction, but its effect is as devastating as that of cocaine or alcohol. Many people lose their home, their family, their identity. Some end up in prison. Others end up dead. The worst thing is that most do not ask for help in time due to shame, denial or because "it is not a drug".

5.1.8 Gambling in History and Art

- Fyodor Dostoevsky wrote The Gambler inspired by his own addiction. His losses led him to sign abusive contracts with his publishers.
- Charles Bukowski, alcoholic writer and gambler, described his compulsion in horse racing.
- Films such as Uncut Gems, The Gambler or Casino show the progressive deterioration of the compulsive gambler.
- Theater: Gorky's The Player portrays the game as a symbol of decadence.
- Painting: Cézanne's The Card Players conveys the silent tension of the game as an internal struggle.

Clinical case

Marcos, 42 years old, bank manager. He started betting "for fun" on online games. In three years, he lost more than 500,000 pesos, mortgaged his parents' house and falsified financial statements. He attempted suicide after losing his job. He entered outpatient treatment with SSRIs, cognitive behavioral therapy, and assistance to Gamblers Anonymous. Today he has not played for 18 months.

5.1.9 Treatment of Gambling Disorder

Pharmacological treatment

- SSRIs (sertraline, escitalopram): for anxiety, depression and obsessiveness.
- Naltrexone: reduces the impulse and craving for the bet.
- Mood stabilizers: useful if there is associated bipolarity.
- Atypical antipsychotics: in case of severe impulsivity or distorted thinking.

Psychotherapy

- Cognitive behavioral therapy (CBT): identification of distortions, impulse management.
- Group therapy (Gamblers Anonymous): peer support, anonymity, testimonials.
- Family psychoeducation: clear boundaries, prevention of codependency, financial control.

Technological interventions

- Spending monitoring and self-limitation apps.
- Online gambling site blockers.
- External device monitoring.

Emotional and Family Consequences

- Breakdown of relationships, isolation, verbal or physical violence.
- Concealment, chronic lying, theft from family members.
- Secondary trauma in children.
- Feelings of shame, unworthiness, and hopelessness.

Help Resources

- Gamblers Anonymous (JA): free groups around the world.
- Public and private centers specialising in behavioural addictions.
- Emotional emergency lines in Mexico, Spain and the United States.

5.1.10 Gambling Addiction Help Resources

Recovery from problem gambling doesn't have to be a lonely path. There are multiple community, clinical, and digital resources that offer free or specialized support for those suffering from this addiction, as well as for their families and caregivers. Here are the most relevant ones internationally and in three key regions: **Mexico**, **Spain** and the **United States**.

5.1.11 Support Groups: Gamblers Anonymous (JA)

What is it?

Gamblers Anonymous is a worldwide organization based on the 12-step model of Alcoholics Anonymous, adapted to gambling addiction.

It does not require diagnosis, payment or formal registration. It is **free, confidential, and without religious or political affiliation**.

How does it help?

- Active listening and peer support.
- Share personal experiences without judgment.
- Daily follow-up, sponsorship and structured recovery.
- In person or by video call in many countries.

International website:
https://www.gamblersanonymous.org

Specific chapters:

- Mexico: http://jugadoresanonimos.org.mx
- Spain: http://jugadoresanonimos.org.es
- United States: https://www.gamblersanonymous.org/ga/

5.1.12 Specialized public and private centers

Behavioral addiction treatment centers offer comprehensive evaluation, individual or group psychotherapy, pharmacotherapy if needed, and family support. Some combine addiction treatment with comorbid mental disorders such as depression, ADHD or bipolar disorder.

In Mexico:

- **Primary Care Centers for Addictions (CAPA)**: Free and distributed throughout the country (through the National Commission against Addictions–CONADIC). Web: https://www.gob.mx/salud/conadic

- **Specialized private clinics** such as Oceánica, Monte Fénix, or centers with comprehensive residential programs.

In Spain:

- **Addiction Care Network** (UNAD) – Public services and NGO with national coverage. Web: https://www.unad.org

- Centers of the **National Plan on Drugs**, coordinated by autonomous communities.

- Private clinics (CITA Centers, Triora, ForumSalut Mental, etc.).

In the United States:

- SAMHSA (Substance Abuse and Mental Health Services Administration): Offers a national database of treatment resources. Web: https://www.samhsa.gov/find-treatment

- Private clinics with dual programs for addiction and mental health (Hazelden Betty Ford, Kaiser Permanente, etc.).

5.1.13 Emotional Hotlines & Free Consultation

When the urge to gamble becomes intolerable, or when a family is facing a crisis, an immediate hotline can save lives.

Mexico:

- **Lifeline (CONADIC)**: 800 911 2000 (24/7)

- Online chat on its official website

Spain:

- **Telephone Against Addictions (ANAR Foundation and Proyecto Hombre)**

900 200 225 – confidential and free of charge

- **Telephone of Hope:** 717 003 717

United States:

- **National Problem Gambling Helpline:** 1-800-522-4700 (24/7)
- **Crisis Text Line:** Send "HELLO" to the 741741
- **988 Suicide & Crisis Lifeline:** for emotional emergencies

5.1.14 Digital Resources and Self-care Apps

- **BetBlocker/Gamban:** free or low-cost blockers to prevent access to online gambling sites.
- **RecoverMe:** app with tracking, cognitive-behavioral tools and connection with therapists.
- **YouTube, podcasts and moderated forums** with testimonials and guides in Spanish and English.

5.1.15 Family Accompaniment and Support Networks

- **Support groups for family members of players:** similar to Al-Anon.
- **Systemic family therapy** in mental health facilities.
- **Schools for parents and prevention workshops** in educational centers.

5.2 Sex and Pornography Addiction

5.2.1 When Desire Becomes a Prision and Pleasure Loses its Face

Few addictions generate as much shame, secrecy, and denial as **sex and pornography addiction**. In a society saturated with erotic stimuli, where the Internet offers unlimited access to sexual content, this addiction spreads quietly –hidden behind closed doors, private tabs and nocturnal commutes.

Many say, "It's not like drugs or alcohol", but the compulsive pursuit of sexual liberation can destroy marriages, careers, self-esteem, and mental health. Addiction is not to sex itself, but to its **dysregulated, compulsive and disconnected form**.

5.2.2 What is Sex and Pornography Addiction?

Sex or pornography addiction is a **behavioral addiction** characterized by **repetitive and compulsive sexual behaviors**, or by the excessive consumption of pornographic content, despite the negative consequences in personal, relational or professional life.

It is not about sexual frequency or taste, but about **loss of control**, **emotional discomfort** and the **inability to stop**, even when you want to do it deeply.

5.2.3 Neurobiology of Sexual Compulsion

- **Dopamine discharge:** Sexual stimuli –especially visual and novel ones– activate the **dopaminergic reward system**, flooding the brain with pleasurable signals.
- **Tolerance:** Over time, more intense or extreme contents are required to achieve the same effect.
- **Reactivity to cues:** As with drugs, certain stimuli (notifications, images, anxiety) can induce strong desires.
- **Inhibition of the prefrontal cortex:** Chronic use reduces self-control —you act on impulse and then regret comes.
- **Withdrawal symptoms:** Irritability, anxiety, insomnia, and dysphoria when trying to quit.

5.2.4 Signs and Symptoms

- Loss of control over time spent on sex or pornography.
- Using sex or masturbation as an escape from stress, sadness, or loneliness.
- Progressive escalation: search for more extreme or risky content.
- Failed attempts to quit.
- Negligence of work, couple, hygiene and responsibilities.
- Guilt, emotional disconnection and emptiness after the act.

5.2.5 Common Triggers

- Emotional stress, loneliness, rejection, conflict.

- History of trauma, sexual abuse, or upbringing with bodily shame.
- Attachment wounds and low self-esteem.
- Early exposure (before the age of 12) to pornographic content.
- Lack of secure relationships or emotional intimacy.

5.2.6 Clinical Types of People with Sexual Addiction

- **The emotional avoider:** uses sex to anesthetize trauma, anxiety, or emptiness.
- **The intensity seeker:** needs novelty, risk and constant stimulation.
- **The obsessive ritualist:** creates strict and repetitive routines (hours of browsing, fixed sequences).
- **The intimacy avoider:** prefers digital stimulation to avoid real contact.
- **The re-enactor of traumatic experiences:** repeats dynamics of abuse, humiliation or internalized violence.

5.2.7 Associated Psychiatric Disorders

- ADHD.
- Bipolar disorder (especially in manic phases).
- Borderline personality disorder.
- Major depression.
- Obsessive-compulsive disorder.
- Substance use disorders (alcohol, cocaine, methamphetamines).

Clinical case

Carlos, 29 years old. He started watching pornography at 11. At first it was occasional. By 24, I spent 4-6 hours a day consuming content. His sexual preferences became increasingly extreme, and he lost inh terest in real relationships. She avoided appointments because of performance anxiety and embarrassment. After a suicide attempt, he entered therapy, was treated with SSRIs and CBT, and joined a support group. Two years later, he reports healthy intimacy, integrated desire, and compassion for himself.

Treatment

1. Psychotherapy

- **Cognitive-behavioral therapy (CBT):** to restructure thoughts, break compulsive patterns.
- **EMDR:** Useful if there is childhood trauma or abuse.
- **Mindfulness and relapse prevention.**
- **Sex and couples therapy:** to rebuild emotional intimacy.
- **Support groups:** break isolation and shame.

2. Medication

- **SSRIs:** to reduce obsessive thoughts and compulsions.
- **Naltrexone:** blocks the reward circuit.
- **Mood stabilizers:** in cases of bipolarity.
- **Antiandrogens** (extreme cases and under strict medical supervision).

3. Digital interventions

- **Accountability software:** (CovenantEyes, EverAccountable).
- **site blockers:** (ColdTurkey, Freedom).
- **Sexual detox communities:** (RebootNation, NoFap).

5.2.8 Emotional and Relational Damage

- Sexual dysfunction with the real partner.
- Emotional betrayal and breach of trust.
- Emotional disconnection, contact anxiety, shame.
- Divided identity: “real self” versus “compulsive self”.
- Pornography-induced erectile dysfunction (PIED).

5.2.9 Reflection in Art, Culture and History

Sex addiction is not a new phenomenon or merely clinical. Throughout history, it has been **a recurring theme in literature,**

cinema, painting, music, and public life, because it touches deep fibers of the human soul: desire, emptiness, power, trauma, shame, and the search for meaning. Art, far from condemning, has been a mirror, a cry and catharsis.

***The Picture of Dorian Gray*, by Oscar Wilde**

In this novel, young Dorian makes a pact to keep his beauty intact as his portrait ages and absorbs the signs of his moral degeneration.

What does it represent?

- The insatiable search for pleasure as an escape from suffering.
- The denial of consequences and the cult of superficial desire.
- The reflection of a covert addiction: the character continues to consume beauty, bodies, emotions... but it is increasingly empty.

Dorian Gray doesn't age on the outside, but his soul rots on the inside.

***Shame*, by Steve McQueen (2011)**

Starring Michael Fassbender, this film portrays the life of a man who is externally successful, but deeply enslaved by his sexual addiction.

What does it show?

- The addict's silent and destructive routine.
- Sex as an emotional anaesthesia and not as a connection.
- Existential loneliness, the inability to love, and chronic shame.

Shame does not judge the character: she accompanies him in his pain, his emptiness, his disconnection.

***Nymphomaniac*, de Lars von Trier (2013)**

Divided into two volumes, the story follows a woman who recounts her compulsive sexual experiences from childhood to adulthood.

What does it contribute?

- A raw, poetic and sometimes cruel look at compulsive sexuality.

- The mixture of trauma, pleasure, pain, guilt and desire for redemption.

- The demystification of the hypersexualized woman as a simple object of pleasure.

The protagonist is not an erotic archetype: she is a wound that beats and bleeds in silence.

Egon Schiele, Austrian Expressionist Painter

Famous for his self-portraits and sexually charged nudes, his work shows crooked bodies, empty eyes, explicit genitality, and raw vulnerability.

What does it express?

- The connection between sexuality, anguish and death.

- The body not as an aesthetic object, but as a vehicle of trauma, desire and isolation.

- A pre-psychoanalytic vision of the fragmented body.

Schiele does not paint eroticism: he paints obsession, broken desire, the body that asks to be seen and saved (figure 25).

Prince, Madonna, Nine Inch Nails, Sexual Obsession Artists

- **Prince:** spiritual sensuality and religious provocation; his music combines ecstasy, pleasure, guilt and redemption.

- **Madonna:** eroticism as a political provocation; from Like a Virgin to Erotica, she addresses sexuality as identity and rebellion.

- **Nine Inch Nails:** industrial darkness, lyrics about violent desire, alienation, body as a battlefield.

In all of them, sex is language: to resist, confess and survive (Figure 26).

Historical and contemporary figures

- **Giacomo Casanova:** not only a symbol of seduction, but an early example of compulsion disguised as gallantry.

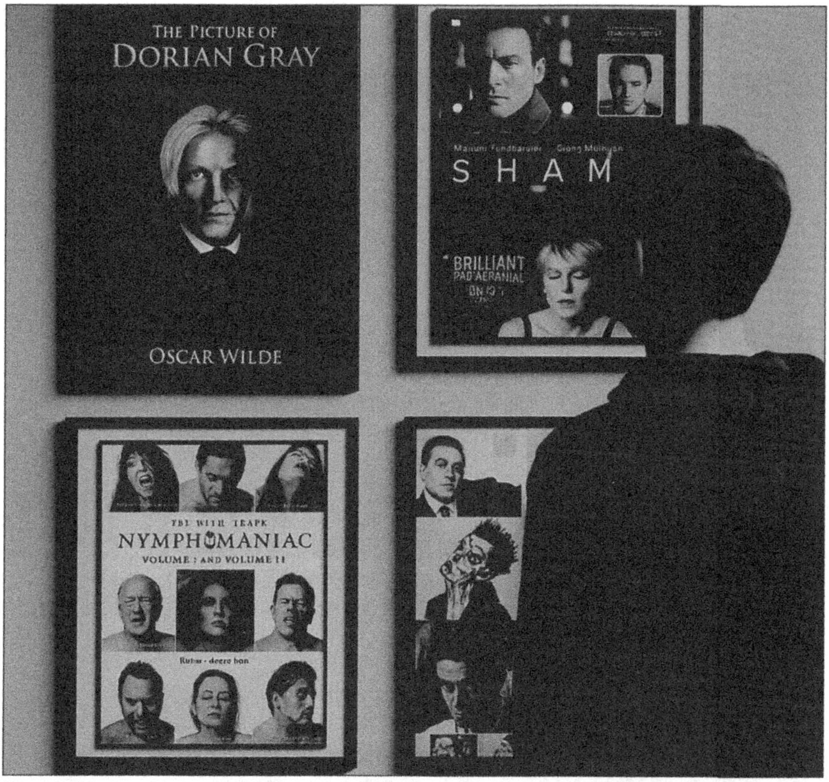

Figure 25. A young man looks at cultural portraits of sexual addiction: from compulsive desire to emotional alienation. The body seeks pleasure, but the mind isolates itself in a cycle that no longer recognizes love.

- **Charlie Sheen:** Actor known for his chaotic lifestyle, multiple relationships, drug use, and public sex scandals.
- **Tiger Woods:** sports idol whose career almost collapsed after the revelation of his sex addiction and his multiple infidelities.

These figures show how sexual addiction does not discriminate against status, talent, or success. Behind the scandal there is usually trauma, emptiness and desperation of real contact (Figure 27).

5.2.10 Help Resources

- Sex Addicts Anonymous (SAA): www.saa-recovery.org

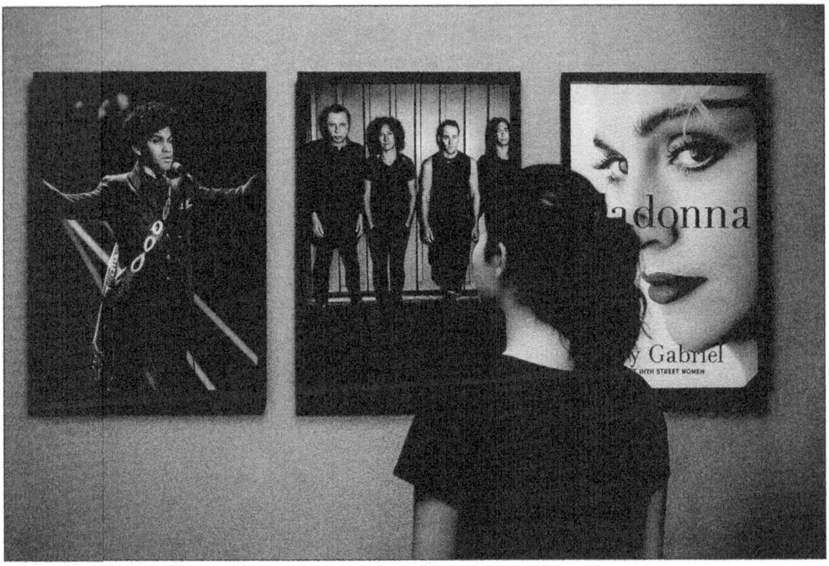

Figure 26. A young woman gazes at pop culture icons whose work explores sexual obsession and unbridled desire. Music reveals what society silences: eroticism as escape, power or addiction.

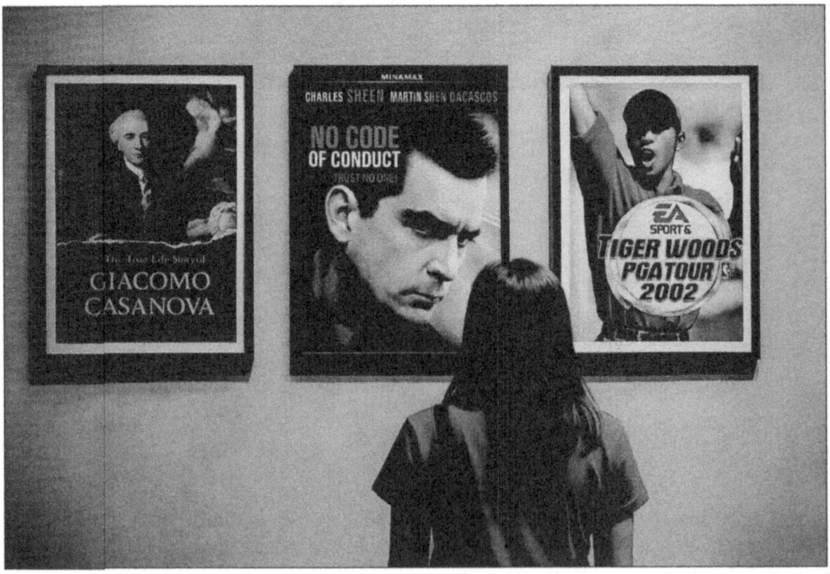

Figure 27. A young woman observes portraits of public figures caught in the spiral of sexual addiction: Casanova, Sheen and Tiger Woods reveal how desire can disguise itself as success, fame or romanticism, but hides patterns of compulsion and self-destruction.

- Love and Sex Addicts (SLAA): www.slaafws.org
- RebootNation/NoFap: Detox Forums and Programs.
- Professional Therapy with Certified Therapists (CSAT).
- Available in **Mexico, Spain and the United States**, in person and virtually.

Help Resources for Sex Addiction and Pornography

Recovery from sexual addiction is not only possible, but **requires structured, safe, and judgment-free support** (Figure 28). Below are the main resources available, from free support groups to certified professionals, with face-to-face and virtual access in **Mexico, Spain** and the**United States.**

1. Sex Addicts Anonymous (SAA)

Official site: www.saa-recovery.org

What is it?

SAA is an international community of people seeking recovery from sexual addiction in all its forms. Their approach is anonymous, free, based on the 12 steps, and is based on mutual support and progressive abstinence.

Features:

- Face-to-face, Zoom, telephone and email meetings.
- No diagnosis or official registration is required.
- Absolute respect for sexual and gender diversity.
- Recovery manuals and guides accessible online.
- Spanish translation available in many groups.

In Mexico, Spain and the United States:

Daily meetings are found in major cities and online for those living in areas without physical groups.

2. Love and Sex Addicts Anonymous (SLAA)

Official site: www.slaafws.org

What is it?

SLAA offers a therapeutic space for people whose sexual compulsion is combined with dysfunctional relationships, emotional dependence, idealization of romantic love, or inability to sustain stable bonds.

Types of addiction addressed:

- Sexual compulsion.
- Compulsive promiscuity.
- Obsessive fantasies.
- Emotional dependence and fear of abandonment.
- Toxic or repetitive relationships.

Program Benefits:

- Comprehensive approach: addresses both sexual addiction and dysfunctional attachment patterns.
- Accompaniment by godparents.
- Work on steps and tools for the management of desire.

Available in Spanish:

Many groups offer meetings in Spanish on all continents. There are virtual meetings adapted to different time zones.

3. Digital Detox Platforms: RebootNation and NoFap

- **RebootNation** (www.rebootnation.org): global community of people seeking freedom from compulsive pornography consumption and healing their sex and emotional lives.
- **NoFap** (www.nofap.com): English-speaking forum with thousands of users, daily challenges, testimonials and practical tips to "reset" the brain reward system.

What they offer:

- Moderate, anonymous and empathetic forums.
- Neuroscientific information on porn addiction.
- Personal and community follow-up (e.g. 30, 60, 90-day challenges).
- Support for single people or couples.
- Payment programs with certified therapists (optional).

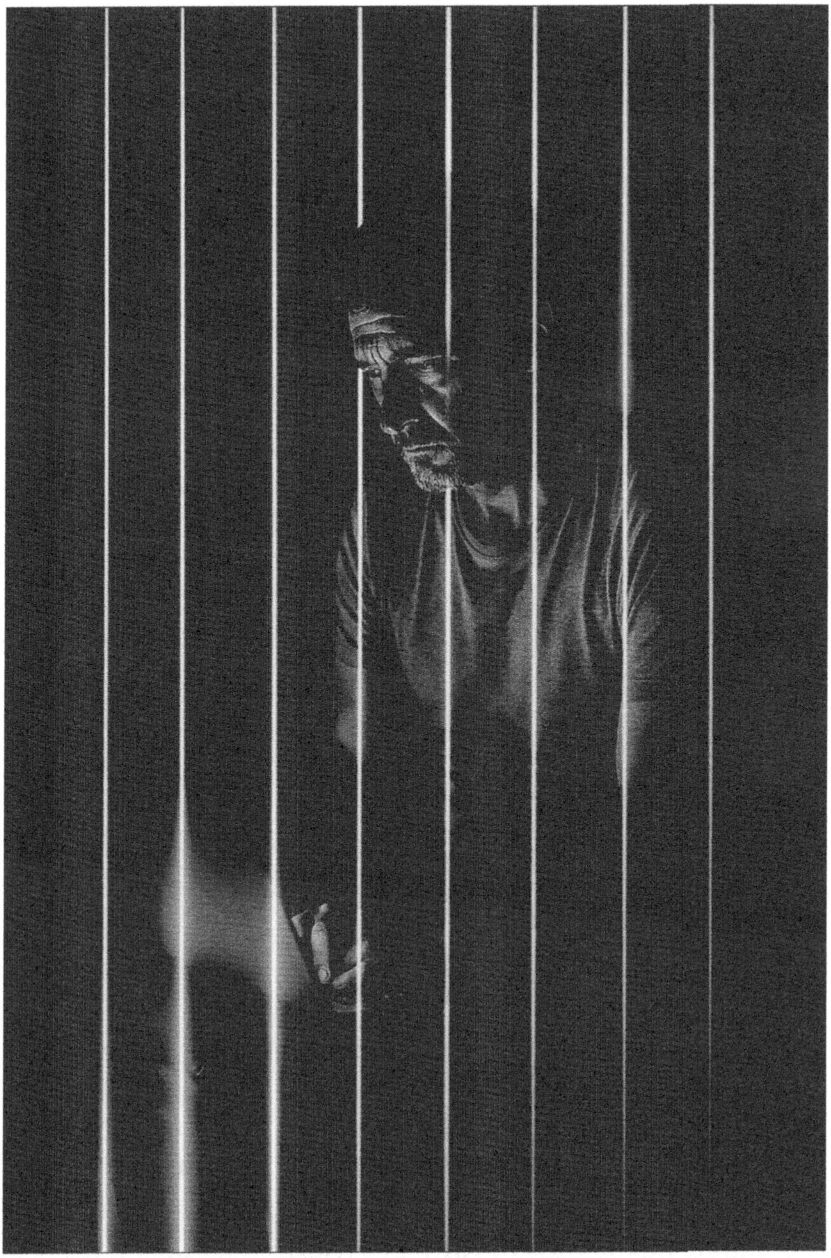

Figure 28. A man trapped in the darkness of his room, lit only by the screen of his laptop, represents addiction to sex and digital pornography. The vertical lines of light suggest a symbolic prison: the invisible bars of compulsive desire and emotional loneliness.

Caution:

Although they are useful as a complement, they do not replace professional clinical or psychotherapeutic accompaniment. Their content needs to be critically reviewed, as some communities may have rigid ideological approaches.

4. Professional Therapy with Certified Therapists (CSAT)

What is a CSAT therapist?

The Certified Sex Addiction Therapist is a professional trained by Dr. Patrick Carnes and the International Institute for Trauma and Addiction Professionals (IITAP).

Benefits of working with a CSAT:

- Professional assessment of the level of addiction.
- Intervention with a scientific basis, without moralism or judgment.
- Inclusion of underlying trauma, shame, and attachment patterns.
- Integration with couple, family and other therapies.
- Personalized recovery plan.

How to find them?

- www.iitap.com: allows you to search for therapists by country, city and modality (virtual/face-to-face).
- In **Mexico**, CSATs exist in Mexico City, Guadalajara, and Monterrey.
- In **Spain**, some therapists are trained in parallel models (ITAM, CTT).
- In the **United States** there are hundreds of therapists with official credentials, both in private centers and online platforms.

5. Local and Online Access in Mexico, Spain, and the United States

In Mexico:

- **Public mental health clinics of** INSABI and the Ministry of Health.

- **Fray Bernardino Álvarez Psychiatric Hospital** (CDMX): specialized care in addictions and sexual health.

- **Comprehensive private centers** such as Monte Fénix, Oceánica, Camino a Casa, which integrate sexual and couple therapy.

In Spain:

- **Public centers of the National Plan on Drugs.**

- **Clinics specialising** in compulsive sexual behaviour: Triora, Forum Mental Health, etc.

- **UNAD (Addiction Care Network):** with a presence in almost all the autonomous communities.

In the United States:

- **SAMHSA** – National Database of Addiction and Mental Health Centers (www.samhsa.gov/find-treatment)

- **TherapyDen/PsychologyToday:** Directories to search for CSATs, clinical sexologists, groups, and bilingual therapists.

- **Telemedicine programs** with access to psychiatrists, therapists, and virtual groups.

5.3 Addiction to Technology, Social Media, and Video Games

5.3.1 When the Mind Slips Non-stop and the Soul Disconects from the Present

We live in an era of hyperconnectivity. Never before has humanity had immediate access to so many images, messages, rewards, notifications and stimuli. But that abundance has also generated a **new form of silent dependence**, fueled by algorithms, dopamine, and existential emptiness: addiction to digital devices.

This form of addiction is not injected, smoked, or drunk. **It is swiped with the finger**, **shared**, **commented on**, **consumed in secret or even in public**. And yet, it can be as devastating as any drug.

5.3.2 What is Technology Addiction?

Technology addiction is an **impulse control disorder** characterized by the compulsive use of digital devices —such as phones, video games, social networks, or web browsing —that significantly interferes with personal, school, work, family, or emotional life.

Not all heavy use is addictive. The problem arises when you **lose control**, when technology becomes an **emotional drain**, and when everything else begins to deteriorate.

5.3.3 Neurobiology of Digital Addiction

- **Dopamine:** Social media and video games stimulate the dopaminergic system with likes, virtual rewards, quick achievements, and intermittent stimuli.
- **Variable reward circuit:** Like slots, technology offers unpredictable rewards that reinforce compulsion (likes, messages, prizes).
- **Emotional dysregulation:** By avoiding boredom, sadness or anxiety through screens, the brain stops developing tolerance to discomfort.
- **Hypersensitivity to digital stimuli** and **hypoactivity of the prefrontal cortex** in adolescents with overuse.

5.3.3.1Types of Technology Addiction

1- Social media (Instagram, TikTok, X/Twitter, Facebook, etc.)

- Compulsive search for validation, social comparison, rapid dopamine.- Anxiety about likes, FOMO (fear of missing out), and need for exposure.

2- Video games (online, consoles, mobiles)

- Increased tolerance: hours of play, economic expense, isolation.
- Games with addictive design: rewards, levels, challenges and purchase of content.
- Effects: insomnia, aggressiveness, difficulty concentrating, avoidance of real relationships.

3- Addiction to scrolling or infinite navigation

- YouTube, Reddit, news, forums, etc.
- Passive trance state, extreme procrastination, fragmentation of attention.

4- Nomophobia and cell phone dependence

- Anguish when forgetting the phone, checking notifications every few minutes.
- Physical symptoms if there is no signal or battery: sweating, irritability, panic.

5.3.4 How is it Diagnosed?

There is still no universal consensus to classify this addiction as a formal disorder (except for **video game addiction**, recognized by the World Health Organization since 2019), but the following criteria are useful:

- Prolonged, compulsive use, with loss of control.
- Discomfort or anxiety when trying to limit use.
- Progressive social isolation.
- Impairment of sleep, school/work performance, food and relationships.
- Use as an emotional escape: to not feel or not face situations.

Clinical case

Erick, 16 years old, started playing video games 1 hour a day. In a year, I spent up to 10 hours a day online. He quit the sport, stopped hanging out with friends, and his grades dropped dramatically. When he tried to take away his access, he reacted with anger and even physical aggression. He was diagnosed with video game addiction and mild depression. She is currently in family therapy and under treatment with sertraline.

5.3.5 Short- and Long-term Consequences

In children and adolescents:

- Delay in social skills, insomnia, sedentary lifestyle, irritability.
- Increased anxiety, aggressiveness, poor academic performance.
- Greater vulnerability to bullying, grooming and digital violence.

In adults:

- Chronic procrastination, loss of productivity, loneliness.
- Relationship problems, lack of real intimacy, emotional dissociation.
- Visual fatigue, insomnia, mood alteration.

Treatment:

1. Individual and Family Psychotherapy

- Cognitive behavioral therapy (CBT): regulation of use, impulse management.
- Controlled exposure therapy for use.
- Mindfulness, emotional regulation, reinforcement of social skills.
- Family therapy: establishment of rules, limits and accompaniment.

2. Structured Digital Intervention

- Blocking apps, parental control, defined schedules.
- Usage monitoring with agreements and follow-up.
- Progressive replacement by non-digital recreational activities.

3. Pharmacological Treatment (when there is Comorbidity)

- SSRIs: anxiety, depression, irritability.
- Mood stabilizers: severe impulsivity.
- Medication in ADHD if there are comorbid symptoms.

5.3.6 Culture, Art and Social Criticism

Technology addiction has not only become a clinical and social challenge, but also a profound source of artistic and critical reflection on the modern world:

***Black Mirror* (series)**: Dystopian anthology that explores humanity's dark relationship with technology. Each episode functions as a warning about how uncontrolled digital progress can lead to isolation, loss of autonomy, and dehumanization.

***Ready Player* One (novel/film)**: Depicts a society where real life is so unbearable that people escape into a hyper-stimulating virtual reality world. The story reflects the risks of digital escapism and the consequences of leaving the physical world.

***Edward Hopper* (painter)**: His solitary figures looking out the window or surrounded by empty spaces capture the emotional alienation and disconnection of the modern individual, a theme that resonates with the overuse of the digital.

***Her* (Spike Jonze film)**: Tells the story of a man who falls in love with an artificial intelligence. It questions what constitutes real intimacy, the limits of emotional substitution through technology, and our growing reliance on artificial connections.

***The Social Dilemma* (documentary)**: Offers a hard-hitting critique of how tech companies manipulate user behavior using algorithms and dopamine loops, directly contributing to addiction, polarization, and deteriorating mental health.

These works act as cultural mirrors, warning us about the potential emotional and existential costs of our digital obsessions (Figure 29).

5.3.7 Help Resources

- Ciberadicciones.com: Psychologists specialized in digital addiction. **(Mexico/Spain)**
- Common Sense Media: Resources for parents, teachers, and youth.
- Digital Addiction Institute (IDDA): Behavioral intervention programs.
- World Health Organization: Diagnostic Manual for Video Game Addiction.

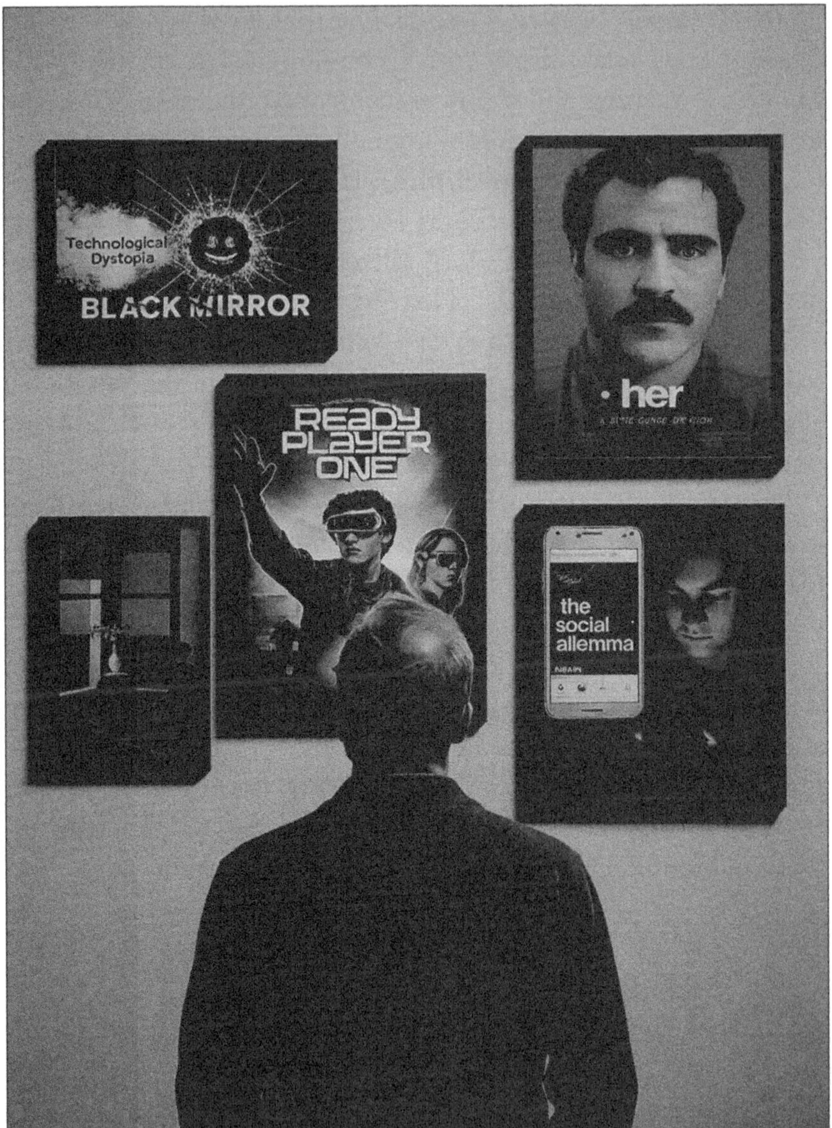

Figure 29. A man looks at a symbolic gallery of works exploring the impact of technology addiction. From the digital dystopia of Black Mirror, to the escape in Ready Player One and the intimate loneliness of Her, to the paintings of Edward Hopper and the documentary The Social Dilemma, this composition denounces how technology can distort our emotions, bonds and sense of reality.

- Psychological support lines and digital guidance in mental health hospitals

Recovery from a technological addiction requires both personal awareness and access to adequate resources. Below are platforms, organizations, and specialized spaces –face-to-face and virtual– that offer clinical, educational, and community help, available in **Mexico**, **Spain**, the **United States**, and online.

1. Ciberadicciones.com

Focus: specialized psychotherapy for digital addictions, video games, social networks and technology in young people and adults.

Features:

- Certified professionals in technology psychology.
- Programs for children, teens, adults, and families.
- Individual, group, and family therapy (face-to-face and online).
- Clinical diagnosis, psychological reports, prevention workshops.
- With a presence in Mexico City, Guadalajara, Monterrey and remote modality for all of Latin America and Spain.

2. CommonSense Media

Focus: Safe digital education for parents, teachers, and students.

Features:

- Recommendations for digital use by age and school stage.
- Reviews of video games, apps, movies and platforms with a pedagogical approach.
- Free guides on screen limits, addiction, cyberbullying, and digital privacy.
- Workshops and school resources in English and Spanish.
- Widely used in schools in the United States, Spain, and Latin America.

3. Digital Addiction Institute (IDDA)

Focus: behavioral intervention and clinical treatment of technological addictions.

Features:

- Founded by experts in neuropsychiatry and digital addictive behavior.
- Neuropsychological evaluation of severity of addiction to video games, digital pornography, social networks.
- Intensive behavioral interventions (virtual and face-to-face).
- Family therapy and personalized digital detox plans.
- Programs with scientific evidence and certified protocols.
- Headquarters in the United States, with international expansion and video call therapy.

4. World Health Organization (WHO)

Approach: standardization and recognition of video game addiction as a clinical disorder.

Features:

- Since 2019, Gaming Disorder has been included in ICD-11.
- Official diagnostic criteria for mental health professionals.
- Promotion of public health strategies and preventive education.
- Resources for governments and health systems on how to address this emerging issue.

Access: www.who.int

5. Psychological Support and Digital Guidance Lines

Mexico:

- **SAPTEL** (800 472 7835): 24/7 emotional care, free of charge, with trained psychologists.
- **IMSS Psychological Well-being:** appointments with mental health specialists with a digital approach.

- **UNAM and Tec de Monterrey:** university clinics with care for technological addiction.

Spain:

- **ANAR Foundation** (900 202 010): psychological help for children and adolescents.
- **Telephone of Hope** (717 003 717): emotional guidance and crisis.
- **Public mental health centers** of the National Health System.

United States:

- **SAMHSA Helpline** (1-800-662-HELP): Toll-free, confidential, 24/7.
- **PsychologyToday:** search engine for therapists with experience in digital addictions.
- **Teen Line and Crisis Text Line:** specialized care for young people with digital anxiety and isolation.

Complementary platforms and apps:

- **Forest:** helps limit cell phone use through visual ecological dynamics.
- **Freedom:** blocks sites and apps for defined hours.
- **Moment:** Analyzes phone usage time with daily statistics.
- **Opal:** applies conscious focusing techniques and notification management.

5.4 Shopping Addiction and Impulse Control Disorders

5.4.1 When the Desire to Buy Becomes an Escape Mechanism

Shopping addiction —also known as oniomania— is not simply about spending too much, but an impulsive-compulsive disorder where shopping acts as temporary relief from painful emotions such as anxiety, emptiness, stress or loneliness. This urge becomes repetitive, self-destructive, and difficult to stop behavior, even when there are serious financial, family, or personal consequences.

Clinical Features

- Obsessive thoughts about products, offers, or pending purchases.
- Feeling euphoric or relieved when shopping, followed by guilt or shame.
- Accumulation of unnecessary objects, often unopened.
- Lies to hide purchases or debts.
- Significant interference in personal, work, or family relationships.

It is frequently associated with disorders such as depression, anxiety, bipolar disorder, ADHD, and personality disorders (such as borderline or narcissistic).

5.4.2 Neurobiology of Impulse

Like other behavioral addictions, shopping addiction activates the **dopaminergic reward circuit**, especially the nucleus accumbens and the prefrontal cortex. Immediate gratification clouds the ability to reflect, and anticipation of the act of buying stimulates the release of dopamine.

Over time, **emotional tolerance is created** –spending more is required to get the same relief. And emotional withdrawal can lead to symptoms such as irritability, anxiety, or existential emptiness.

5.4.3 Risk Factors

- Childhood marked by affective or material deficiencies.
- Cultures focused on consumption as a way of identity and belonging.
- Low self-esteem and need for external validation.
- Mood disorders or previous traumatic experiences.
- Continuous exposure to social media, advertising, and aspirational lifestyles.

5.4.4 Treatments

1. Cognitive-behavioral Psychotherapy (CBT):

It helps identify distorted thoughts, emotional patterns, and replace compulsive behavior with healthy strategies.

2. Third wave therapies:

Such as Dialectical-Behavioural Therapy or mindfulness, useful in patients with high impulsivity or comorbidities.

3. Family or couples therapy:

Essential when there are economic or relational problems due to addiction.

4. Medication:

SSRIs (such as fluoxetine or sertraline) in cases of comorbidity with depression or OCD. Mood stabilizers in bipolar patients.

5. Group treatments:

- Debtors Anonymous (DA)
- Compulsive Shoppers Anonymous (CCA)

5.4.5 Reflections in Culture and Art

The compulsive need to buy, consume and possess has been the subject of profound critical reflection in film, television, literature and the visual arts. These works not only show shopping as a superficial act, but reveal emotional, psychological, and social wounds behind materialism (figure 30).

***Confessions of a Compulsive Shopper* (2009)**

Although it is presented as a romantic comedy, this film offers a powerful emotional insight into the inner torment of someone struggling with a shopping addiction. The protagonist, Rebecca Bloomwood, lives under the illusion of control and beauty through luxury goods, while her emotional world collapses. It reflects the progressive spiral of denial, financial chaos, and shame, and culminates in a redemption that emulates the royal path of many people in recovery.

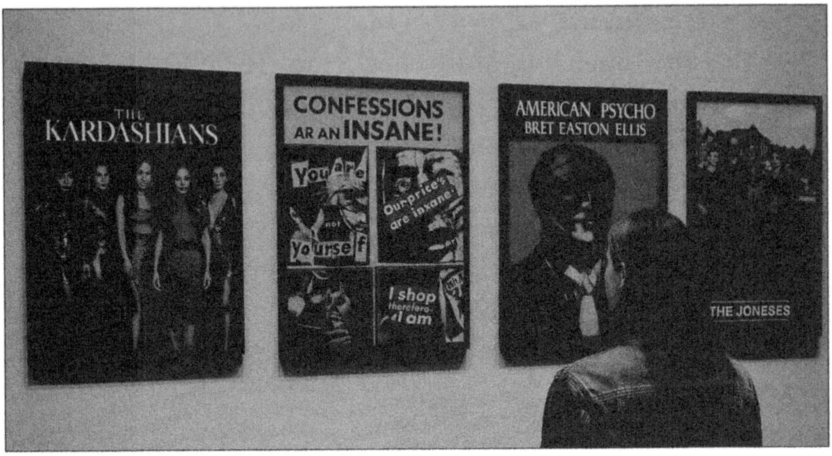

Figure 30. A young woman observes a wall with cultural icons that criticize consumerism and shopping addiction. From the aspirational glamour of Keeping Up with the Kardashians, the capitalist satire of The Joneses and American Psycho, to the provocative artistry of Barbara Kruger and the comedic confession of a compulsive shopper, the image reveals how the desire to possess hides deeper wounds of emptiness, identity and belonging.

***The Joneses* (2009)**

A satirical and sharp critique of consumerist society. The film follows a fake "perfect family" hired to promote luxury goods in a wealthy neighborhood. It dismantles the invisible mechanisms of aspirational marketing, artificial status, and the emotional bankruptcy of appearances. It is a metaphor for how addiction to consumption is socially encouraged and designed by corporations.

***Keeping Up with the Kardashians* (2007–2021)**

This reality show became an international cultural phenomenon by being based on the hyper-consumption of fashion, beauty and lifestyle. It normalized the idea that personal value is measured by what is owned, displayed, and published, influencing millions of people to seek validation through their purchases. For many, it generated an unattainable ideal of success, leading to frustration, comparison, and compulsive behaviors.

Barbara Kruger

American conceptual artist who has masterfully deconstructed the language of advertising, seduction, and identity. Her works –composed of black and white images superimposed with red and white texts– confront the viewer with the manipulative mechanisms of capitalism and gender consumption. Works such as I buy, therefore I exist or Your comfort is my silence are emblems of the emotional void that consumption tries to fill.

***American Psycho, by Bret Easton Ellis* (1991)**

A brutal satire of the yuppie culture of the 80s. It tells the story of Patrick Bateman, a banker obsessed with brands, status and appearances, who is immersed in violence and emotional emptiness. It presents consumption as dehumanization, where the identity of the protagonist is completely defined by what he wears, owns and devours. The novel explores the dark psychological landscape of a world where shopping is a mask for loneliness, disconnection, and moral decay.

5.4.6 Help Resources

Shopping addiction, although often minimized or misunderstood, requires serious clinical and therapeutic accompaniment. There are international and local resources that provide support, treatment, and community:

- Debtors Anonymous (DA)

Website: www.debtorsanonymous.org

12-Step Recovery Program for people whose lives have been affected by uncontrollable debt and binge drinking. It offers face-to-face and virtual meetings, tools for financial stability and emotional healing.

- Compulsive Shoppers Anonymous (SA)

Website: www.shopaholicsanonymous.org

Support Network for People Struggling with Shopping Addiction. It offers anonymous groups, educational material, and community forums for recovery.

Clinics and Therapeutic Centers

Mexico

- Clínica Santa Catalina (CDMX)–Programs specialized in impulse control disorders.
- Psychoaddictions Mexico–Multidisciplinary approach with CBT, mindfulness and family therapy.

Spain

- Institute of Advanced Psychology (Madrid)–Treatment of oniomania and financial dependence.
- Adana Foundation (Barcelona)–Behavioral health care, including non-substance addictions.

United States

- Behavioral Addictions Clinic–UCLA
- The Center for Internet and Technology Addiction–Connecticut.

Online Therapy Platforms

- BetterHelp and Talkspace: Connect patients with therapists who specialize in compulsive behaviors.
- Online Psychology (Spanish-speaking): Certified clinical psychologists with experience in shopping addiction.
- Some platforms include financial planning tools, expense tracking apps, and economic recovery coaching.

5.5 Workaholism

5.5.1 When Productivity Becomes a Prison

Workaholism –known clinically as **workaholism**– is one of the most normalized and socially rewarded behavioral addictions. Apparently, it is associated with success, discipline and ambition. But at its core it hides a pattern of compulsion, emotional evasion, relational deterioration and deep physical and mental exhaustion. Unlike healthy work commitment, the workaholic does not work out of passion, but out **of an internal need for control, achievement or validation**, often unconscious.

5.5.2 Clinical Features

- Constant need to work even outside of hours or rest days.
- Feeling of guilt or anxiety at not producing.
- Difficulty mentally and emotionally disconnecting from work.
- Neglect of personal relationships, sleep, physical health, and overall well-being.
- Denial of the problem, minimization or justification under ideas such as "I like my job" or "I am a perfectionist".

Workaholism can coexist with generalized anxiety, obsessive-compulsive disorders, covert depression, unprocessed trauma, or a personality disorder.

5.5.3 Neuropsychological Basis

Compulsive work sustainably activates the brain's reward circuit, with repeated release of dopamine and cortisol. The feeling of accomplishment, praise, or control activates the nucleus accumbens and amygdala, creating a psychological addiction to productivity. This leads to progressive self-exploitation, similar to other forms of non-substance addiction.

Over time, the body enters into chronic hyperactivation of the HPA (hypothalamus–pituitary–adrenal axis), which generates insomnia, persistent fatigue, digestive, cardiovascular and affective problems.

5.5.4 Causes and Risk Factors

- Childhoods with love conditioned on performance ("I'm worth it if I do").
- Perfectionist or emotionally absent parents.
- Social models that glorify burnout and material success.
- Low self-esteem sustained by external achievements.
- Financial insecurity or fear of failure.
- Toxic, competitive or limitless work cultures.

5.5.5 Treatment and Recovery

1. Individual Psychotherapy:

- CBT: identification of rigid beliefs such as "if I rest, I am useless".

- Psychodynamic therapy: exploring childhood wounds or overcompensating structures.

- Compassion therapy or mindfulness to reconnect with the present and self-care.

2. Couples or Family Therapy:

- Restore bonds, limits and affective roles damaged by the emotional absence of the workaholic.

3. Organizational Intervention (when Applicable):

- Coaching, task redesign, evaluation of work environments and prevention of burnout.

4. Meditation, Scheduled Rest, and Intentional Non-Productive Activities:

- Conscious leisure exercises.

- Reconnection with art, nature, play, creativity and non-instrumental links.

5.6 Reflections in Culture and Art

The figure of the workaholic has been critically portrayed in film, literature, visual art, and television, not as a hero of effort, but as someone who sacrifices his identity, his bonds, and his well-being on the altar of performance.

***The Devil Wears Fashion* (2006)–Dir. David Frankel**

This modern comedy-drama follows a young assistant in the fashion industry, who rises quickly at the cost of her time, her relationships, her values, and her personal freedom. The film shows **emotional servitude disguised as opportunity**, and poses the question: How much of your soul are you willing to trade for professional prestige? Its strength lies in exposing how **corporate culture manipulates ambition into silent obedience**, and how personal value is tied to the approval of power figures.

***Up in the Air* (2009)–Dir. Jason Reitman**

This film explores **emotional disconnection disguised as hyperproductivity**. The protagonist, an executive specializing in layoffs, spends his life flying from city to city, and boasts of his independence and minimalist lifestyle. But beneath that apparent freedom there is a **deep existential emptiness**: no community, no roots, no real intimacy. It is a metaphor for the modern professional who confuses movement with meaning, and distance with strength.

***The Fatigue Society*–Byung-Chul Han**

In this short but powerful philosophical essay, the Korean-German thinker Byung-Chul Han argues that today we live in a society where **exploitation no longer comes from others, but from oneself**. The individual becomes **master and slave at the same time**, constantly pushing himself to perform more, optimize more, excel more. This **silent self-exploitation** generates anxiety, isolation and exhaustion, not because we are forced to, but because we believe that to rest is to fail.

M.C. Escher

Escher's impossible structures and infinite stairs are a disturbing metaphor for the **mental architecture of the workaholic**: always climbing, but not getting anywhere. Each corridor leads to another task, each door to another commitment. Pattern repetition mirrors cognitive loops, where the mind gets caught in a **maze of meaningless productivity**.

Fictional Workaholic Characters

- **Mr. Banks** (Mary Poppins): A bank clerk so absorbed in his formal role that he forgets to play with his children or feel joy. Only when her world collapses, does she rediscover love and balance.

- **Walter White** (Breaking Bad): At first, a man who only wanted to secure the future of his family, Walter becomes addicted not only to his illegal work, but to the **power, identity and control it gives him**. Her moral decay grows as she works harder, showing how overwork can **erase values**, humanity, **and real connection**.

These works are **cultural mirrors** that reveal the high **psychospiritual cost** of a society that equates productivity with virtue (Figure 31).

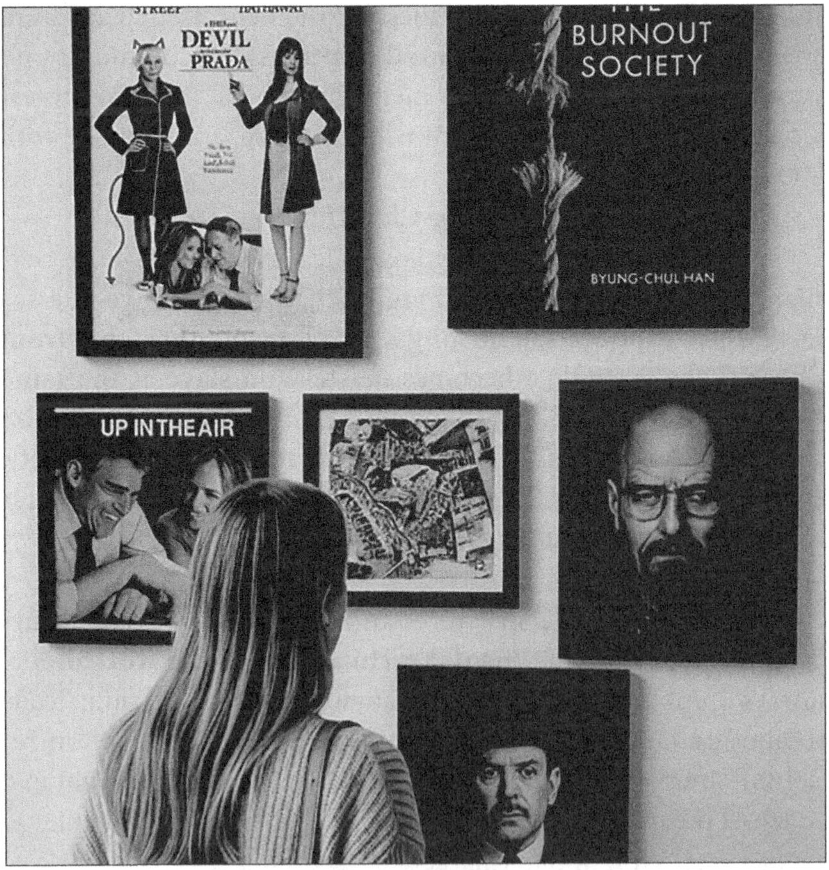

Figure 31. A young woman contemplates a wall illustrating the figure of the workaholic in contemporary culture. From the exhausting perfectionism of The Devil Wears Fashion, the corporate loneliness of Up in the Air, the philosophical analysis of The Fatigue Society, to the emotional rigidity of Mr. Banks and the dangerous transformation of Walter White, the image denounces how the cult of productivity can erase the soul, relationships, and meaning of life.

5.6.1 Help Resources

Overcoming workaholism requires more than resting: it involves rebuilding identity, values, and boundaries. Below are specialized resources available internationally:

Workaholics Anonymous (WA)

www.workaholics-anonymous.org

12-Step Recovery Fellowship for People Who Work Compulsively. It offers face-to-face and virtual meetings, supporting literature, and a spiritual model of healing based on honesty, surrender, and balance.

Behavioral Addiction Clinics

Mexico

- CITA Mexico Clinic (CDMX): specialized in compulsive behaviors and executive burnout.
- Integral Therapy (Guadalajara): intervention with CBT and mindfulness.

Spain

- Therapeutic Institute of Behavioral Addictions (Madrid).
- Centro Aesthesis (Barcelona): personalised programmes for work anxiety and perfectionism.

United States

- The Center for Internet and Technology Addiction (Connecticut).
- MenningerClinic (Houston) – programs for high-performing professionals.

Digital detox and corporate disconnect retreats

Programs such as **Unplugged, Digital Detox Retreats** or **The Stillness Project** offer immersive experiences in nature designed to break workaholism and hyperconnectivity. Many include therapeutic sessions, yoga, silence, writing, and personal reconnection.

Coaching and emotional rebalancing platforms

- **Better Up, Noom Mental Fitness, Mindshine**: applications and mobile platforms that combine emotional coaching, cognitive tools and support systems for those looking to work less and live longer.

- **Balance by Nature** (United States): corporate wellness programs that transform organizational culture to prevent burnout.

Recommended books for recovery and self-knowledge

- *Rest: Why You Do More WhenYou Work Less*–Alex Soojung-Kim Pang.

He maintains that rest is not passivity, but the key to creativity and health.

- *Chained tothe Desk*–Bryan E. Robinson Ultimate psychological guide to understanding and healing workaholism.

- *Driven to Distraction at Work*–Edward M. Hallowell explore how distraction, anxiety, and perfectionism fuel overwork and how to regain attention and presence.

5.7 Food Addiction and Compulsive Eating

5.7.1 When Comfort Becomes Prison

Food addiction is not simply a problem of will. It is a complex disorder that involves brain circuits of reward, emotional regulation, trauma, culture, and deeply ingrained habits. It is not physiological hunger, but an emotional appetite that is not satiated with nutrients, but with meaning.

5.7.2 Definition and Diagnosis

Food addiction can include:

- Recurrent binge eating, even in the absence of hunger.
- Feelings of guilt, shame or hopelessness after eating.
- Loss of control over certain foods, especially ultra-processed foods.
- Need to eat to calm emotions (anger, sadness, anxiety).

It is frequently associated with b**inge eating disorder (BED)**, mood disorders, childhood trauma, and obesity.

5.7.3 Neurobiology Involved

- Excessive activation of the reward circuit (dopamine, nucleus accumbens).
- Ultra-processed foods rich in sugars and fats activate these circuits just like drugs.
- Leptin and insulin resistance: the brain does not "register" satiety.
- Dysregulation of serotonin and the hypothalamic-pituitary-adrenal (HPA) axis, with a greater response to stress.

5.7.4 Root Causes

- Childhood marked by emotional neglect or use of food as a reward or comfort.
- Family models where eating replaces the emotional bond.
- Unverbalized emotional trauma that manifests itself in silent binge eating.
- Food as the only source of pleasure, control or predictability.

5.7.5 Physical and Psychological Consequences

- Obesity, hypertension, dyslipidemia, insulin resistance, sleep apnea.
- Depression, anxiety, social isolation, low self-esteem.
- Cycles of severe restriction and overeating.
- Functional gastrointestinal disorders.

5.7.6 Comprehensive Treatment

- **Cognitive-behavioral therapy specialized** in eating disorders.
- **Support groups** such as Overeaters Anonymous (OA).
- **Psychodynamic psychotherapy** to address trauma and emotional emptiness.
- **Nutritional therapy without restrictive diets**, based on mindful eating.
- Medication in selected cases: antidepressants, naltrexone-bupropion, topiramate.

5.7.7 Reflections in Culture and Art

Food addictions and the compulsive relationship with food are not only explored in the clinic or in psychology, but have been deeply reflected in art, film, literature, and music as symbols of a broader malaise: emotional pain, alienation, abundance as emptiness, and the body as a cultural battlefield (Figure 32).

***The Whale* (2022)**

Directed by Darren Aronofsky and starring Brendan Fraser, this film presents a morbidly obese English teacher who lives in isolation, trapped by guilt, grief and food as his only consolation.

The Relevant Thing: The film does not seek to exploit the image of the body, but to show the deep psychic pain that inhabits it. It becomes an allegory of how food can become a refuge, punishment and symbol of accumulated trauma. It is a play about shame, self-destruction and the possibility of redemption through the human bond.

***Hunger*–Contemporary work**

Different contemporary plays (such as those of Sarah Kane or free adaptations of "Hunger" by Knut Hamsun) have dramatized the struggle between desire and repression, showing characters who face physical hunger as a mirror of emotional and existential hunger.

The symbolic: Hunger, both for food and affection, appears as a metaphor for an internal emptiness. The relationship with food becomes a rite of power, self-punishment or denial.

Fernando Botero–Art as Visual Criticism

The Colombian artist is known for his voluminous figures, which far from being mere caricatures, function as a critique of the excesses of consumption, superficiality and social ostentation.

Psychosocial interpretation: In Botero, large bodies can represent both abundance and excess. Pleasure, gluttony, greed, but also tenderness and nostalgia. They are bodies that take up a lot of space because they contain more than fat: they contain history, inequality, criticism and culture.

***Sugar Blues*-William Dufty**

This cult essay written in the 70s denounces refined sugar as an addictive drug covered up by the system. Dufty argues that sugar produces mood swings, dependence, and chronic diseases, with effects similar to those of other banned substances.

Impact: The book marked an awakening about food as addictive agents, and opened the discussion on the role of the food industry in public health and the psychopathology of consumption.

***Foodis Love* and other theme songs**

Songs like Foodis Love or popular lyrics that link food with affection ("I eat because I'm lonely", "Chocolate saves the day") show how in the collective imagination, food not only nourishes the body, but also soothes emotional wounds.

The emotional: Music puts into words what many do not say: that we eat to fill emotional voids. Food replaces love, attention, comfort. And when that becomes a pattern, compulsion is born.

5.7.8 Help Resources

In addition to cultural analysis, it is vital to offer real bridges to treatment and community. Here are some key resources:

Overeaters Anonymous (OA): www.oa.org

An international community based on the 12 steps (Alcoholics Anonymous style), offering support groups for people with binge eating, bulimia, sugar addiction and more.

Advantage: It is free, confidential, and offers spiritual and community tools to break cycles of shame and loneliness.

National Associations for Eating Disorders

- **Mexico:** Mexican Association of Eating Disorders (AMTA): www.amta.org.mx
- **Spain:** Association in Defense of Care for Anorexia Nervosa and Bulimia (ADANER): www.adaner.org
- **United States:** National Eating Disorders Association (NEDA): www.nationaleatingdisorders.org

Why Are They Important?

These organizations offer professional care, educational programs, helplines, family groups, and awareness campaigns about the physical, psychological, and cultural damage of eating disorders.

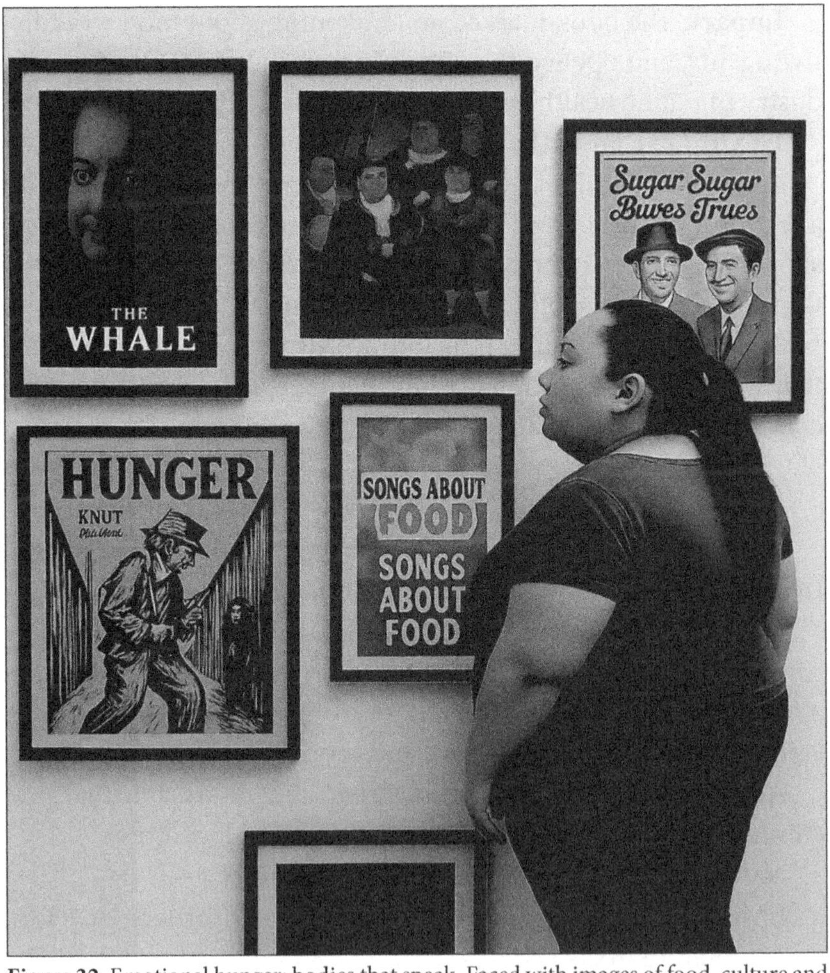

Figure 32. Emotional hunger: bodies that speak. Faced with images of food, culture and the body, a woman silently contemplates the symbolic weight of hunger. It is not only about food, but about what it represents: comfort, absence, tenderness or punishment. From Botero's figures to music about food as love, art reveals that appetite is not always born from the stomach, but from emotional wounds. Eating, sometimes, is an attempt to fill the soul.

CHAPTER 6
Comprehensive Addiction Treatment. Between Science, Psychotherapy and Human Containment

6.1 Diagnostic Assessment and Motivation for Change

The first therapeutic act is to look without fear. The second, to reach out. Evaluating is not just labeling a diagnosis. It is to open a window into the patient's history, their body, their mind, their wounds and their context. In addictions, evaluating involves **recognizing the pain that is hidden behind the symptom.**

Addiction is not only a destructive behavior: it is, many times, **a way of surviving psychic suffering**. The goal is not to judge, but to understand. It is not about classifying, but about finding a starting point.

6.1.1 Dimensions of the Comprehensive Assessment

1. Biomedical Evaluation

- Complete medical history: liver, kidney, neurological damage, associated infections (HIV, hepatitis C).
- Laboratory tests: toxicological tests, liver profile, hormonal tests.
- Evaluation of nutrition and sleep status.
- Evaluation of withdrawal or current intoxication (use of scales such as CIWA for alcohol or COWS for opioids).

2. Psychiatric and Psychological Evaluation

- Diagnosis of comorbidities: depression, anxiety, ADHD, bipolar disorder, PTSD, personality disorders.
- Evaluation of cognitive functioning (alterations due to chronic use).

- Emotional evaluation and bonding (unresolved traumas, grief, dissociation).

3. Functional and Behavioral Assessment

- What is the function of the substance? (anesthesia, stimulation, evasion, belonging).
- What are the triggersfor consumption?
- What are the rituals associated with use?
- What do you lose and what do you gain by consuming?

4. Socio-family Evaluation

- Current support network: do you live alone?, who knows what you consume?, is there violence?
- Childhood history: was there neglect, abuse, abandonment, family chaos?
- Current employment, legal and economic situation.

6.1.2 Stages of Motivation to Change (Prochaska and Di-Clemente Model)

Stage	Clinical Description	Appropriate Intervention
Precontemplation	"I don't have any problems". The patient denies or minimizes.	Empathy, information, not direct confrontation.
Contemplation	"Maybe I do have a problem, but I don't know if I want to change".	Explore ambivalences, validate their doubts.
Preparation	"I want to change, but I'm scared. Where do I start?"	Design a plan, reduce barriers, strengthen self-esteem.
Action	"I'm stopping using, but it's hard for me".	Accompanying, structuring, reinforcing, providing practical tools.
Maintenance	"I have changed, but I fear relapsing".	Relapse prevention, new purposes, community.
Relapse	"I used again". (it is not a stage, but it is part of the process).	Accompaniment without judgment, analysis of causes, resilience.

A patient is not pushed to change. He is accompanied to discover his own motive for doing so.

6.1.3 Motivational Interviewing: the Art of Respectful Dialogue

Motivational interviewing (ME) is a person-centered technique that seeks to awaken **internal motivation** without confrontation. Its principles:

- Open-ended questions.
- Reflective listening.
- Emotional validation.
- Do not confront or impose.
- Encourage self-efficacy ("You can").

Clinical case

Patient: "I don't think I have a serious problem, I only use on weekends". Therapist: "Does it bother you that your family thinks there is a problem?"

Patient: "Yes. They say I've changed a lot".

Therapist: "Do you feel that you have changed?"

Patient: "I guess I didn't lie so much before".

That is the golden moment. The change begins in the crack of doubt.

Common Obstacles in Evaluation

- Shame and guilt.
- Lying and minimization.
- Fear of losing ties or jobs if they reveal the truth.
- Confusion: "Am I sick or am I just weak?"
- Hopelessness: "I've already tried everything..."

The therapist must **hold firmly but warmly**, without infantilizing or aggressing.

Symbolic Image: "the Clean Mirror"

A young man looks at himself in a foggy mirror. At first, he sees only a blurred silhouette. Slowly, wipe the crystal with your sleeve. The features of his face appear... and a forgotten scar. In the background, the figure of a child who observes him from the reflection.

To evaluate is to help the patient see themselves again, without disguises. See their story, not just their addiction.

Technical Resources for the Clinician

- **ASI (Addiction Severity Index)**: comprehensive biopsychosocial assessment questionnaire
- **DAST-10/AUDIT/CAGE**: screening for drugs, alcohol and problematic consumption.
- **SCID-5/MINI/PHQ-9/GAD-7**: diagnostic interviews and comorbidity scales.
- **Motivational interviewing (Miller & Rollnick).**

Conclusion

Evaluation is the first true encounter. Diagnosis is not just a clinical name, it is an emotional and existential map. A good therapist does not seek to confirm their hypotheses, but **to understand the story behind the symptom**. And if a safe space is created, change –although slow– begins to germinate.

"Before you cure someone, ask them if they're willing to give up what makes them sick". Hippocrates

6.2 Treatment Phases: Detoxification, Rehabilitation and Reintegration

Curing an addiction is more than giving up a substance: it is re-inhabiting one's own body, time, and bonds.

Addiction treatment is not linear, nor brief, nor uniform for everyone. It requires successive phases that range from **stopping the immediate damage** to **rebuilding a meaningful life**. Each stage has its own objectives and challenges, and must be approached from a **biopsychosocial, emotional** and **spiritual perspective**.

6.2.1 First phase: Detoxification (Detoxification)

Objective:

Remove the substance from the body and control withdrawal symptoms safely.

Duration:

Between 3 and 14 days, depending on the substance and the patient's physical condition.

Main Components:

- **Constant medical supervision.**
- **Pharmacological management** (e.g., benzodiazepines for alcohol, agonists for opioids).
- **Rest, hydration, correction of imbalances.**
- **Initial psychoeducation and early therapeutic bonding.**

Risks:

- Seizures, delirium tremens, hemodynamic instability (alcohol, benzodiazepines).
- Prolonged withdrawal syndrome (cocaine, marijuana).
- Escape or abandonment attempts.
- Denial, hostility, emotional confusion.

Clinical case

María, 43 years old, arrives at the emergency room after consuming alcohol for 8 days in a row. She is disoriented. He enters the detoxification unit, where he receives thiamine, lorazepam and verbal containment. After 48 hours, she cries: "I didn't remember what it was like to sleep without fear".

6.2.2 Second Phase: Rehabilitation

Objective:

Address the root causes of drug use, relearn coping strategies, and strengthen skills for drug-free living.

Duration:

From 4 weeks to 6 months. It can be outpatient or residential.

Components:

- Individual psychotherapy (CBT, EMDR, psychodynamic therapy).
- Group therapy.
- Training in social and emotional skills.
- Cognitive restructuring and confrontation of addictive beliefs.
- Work with trauma and bonds.
- Life planning and goals.
- Family therapy

Phrases that emerge in this phase:

"I don't know who I am without drugs".

"I use it not to feel. But without use, everything hurts".

"I don't want to fall again, but I don't trust myself".

Clinical case

Luis, 30, has been in a residential center for a month for methamphetamine addiction. During a group session he realizes that he has never cried over the death of his father. That day he does not ask for anxiolytics. For the first time, you feel pain without anesthesia.

6.2.3 Phase Three: Reintegration

Objective:

To return to the social and family environment without relapsing, to build a sustained and healthy life project.

Duration:

Between 3 and 18 months (continuous follow-up). This phase does not have a definitive closing date.

Components:

- Labor or academic reintegration.
- Reestablishment of emotional bonds.
- Relapse prevention (identification of signs, planning).
- Life project: hobbies, spirituality, healthy social networks.

- Psychotherapeutic and medical follow-up.
- Support groups (NA, AA, Al-Anon).

Clinical case

Andrea, 25, a former heroin user, begins to give guitar lessons to children at a cultural center. He says, "I didn't know I had something to give. I thought I only knew how to destroy". That phrase marks the beginning of his reintegration.

6.2.4 Symbolic Image of the Chapter

"The Three-stage Bridge"

A patient walks across a bridge divided into three sections:

- The first, made of old wood, creaks under your feet: it is detoxification.

- The second, made of stone and earth, has signs of bifurcation, shadows and mirrors: it is rehabilitation.

- The third is an open path that crosses a sown field: it is reintegration. In the distance, someone is waiting for him with a light in his hand. It does not guide him. Just accompany him.

Conclusion

Addiction treatment **is not a sprint, but a path of layers and cycles**. There are relapses, setbacks, unexpected advances, and slow awakenings. Not everyone completes all the stages on the first try. But every step taken in awareness **is already part of healing**. Stopping consumption is not enough. We have to learn to live. And then, to love.

6.3 Pharmacological Treatments. Which Medications and When?

It is not enough to remove the poison: the system that housed it must be rebalanced.

6.3.1 Why Pharmacotherapy in Addictions?

Addiction isn't just a choice. It is a neuroadaptive, chronic and relapsing disease. The substances modify receptors, neurotransmitters, and functional networks in the brain. Over time, the following occurs:

- **Hypersensitivity of the reward circuit** (nucleus accumbens, dopamine).
- **Dysregulation of the limbic system** (amygdala, stress, craving).
- **Alteration of the prefrontal cortex** (self-control, judgment, decision-making).
- **Wear and tear of the HPA (hypothalamic-pituitary-adrenal) axis**: chronic anxiety, insomnia, hypervigilance.

Pharmacotherapy, when indicated, **does not seek to "cure" addiction on its own**, but:

- Soften withdrawal.
- Regulate altered neurotransmitters.
- Treat psychiatric comorbidities.
- Reduce craving and impulsivity.
- Create a window of stability for psychotherapy to be effective.

Medications are tools, not solutions. But sometimes, without tools, the process is unfeasible.

6.3.2 General Principles of the Pharmacological Approach

- **Do not replace one addiction with another** (example: be careful with benzodiazepines or stimulants).
- **Evaluate stage of the process**: acute abstinence, post-abstinence, maintenance.
- **Treat comorbidity, not just addiction** (depression, ADHD, anxiety, trauma).
- **Monitor adverse effects, adherence and risk of misuse.**
- **Integrate pharmacotherapy with psychotherapy:** never prescribe without containment.

6.3.3 Treatment According to Type of Substance

A. Alcohol Addiction

1. Neurobiology

- Potentiates GABA-A receptors (inhibitory).
- Blocks NMDA (glutamate, excitatory) receptors.
- Increases dopamine in nucleus accumbens.

2. Phases and medications

Phase	Medication	Main Action	Clinical Commentary
Acute withdrawal	Lorazepam, diazepam, oxazepam	GABAergic, prevent seizures.	Dosage according to CIWA. Controlling sedation.
Maintenance	Acamprosato	Stabilizes glutamate (NMDA).	Reduces craving, useful post-withdrawal.
Maintenance	Oral naltrexone depot	Opioid antagonist, decreases reinforce-ment.	Less pleasure when drinking. Reduces relapses.
Aversion	Disulfiram	Inhibits DH acetaldehyde: generates discomfort if you drink.	Requires adhesion. Risk of toxicity.

Clinical case

Carlos, 52 years old, with 20 years of consumption, achieves abstinence in the center. She reports intense anxiety and fear of relapse. Acamprosate and naltrexone are started. Improved sleep, less craving. At 6 months, he is still abstinent with group support.

B. Opiates: Heroin, Fentanyl, Oxycodone

1. Neurobiology

- Agonism in μ-opioid receptors (analgesia, euphoria).
- Decreased GABA → increased dopamine.
- High tolerance, severe physical dependence.

2. Treatments

Phase	Medication	Action	Observations
Abstinence	Clonidine, Lofexidine	α2-adrenergic agonists → reduce sympathetic activation.	Useful when agonists are not available.
Substitution	Methadone	Complete opioid agonist.	Sets basal level, avoids peaks and withdrawal.
Substitution	Buprenorphine + Naloxone	Partial agonist + antagonist.	Reduced risk of abuse. Requires adhesion.
Blocking	Oral Naltrexone or IM (Vivitrol)	Pure Opioid Antagonist.	Only after complete abstinence. Prevents relapse.

Clinical case

Rosa, 29 years old, IV heroin user. Begins detoxification with buprenorphine under supervision. At 3 weeks, he switches to naltrexone depot. She joins the NA group and receives psychotherapy with a focus on complex trauma.

C. Cocaine and Stimulants (Methamphetamine, Ecstasy)

1. Neurobiology

- Massive increase in dopamine (reuptake block).
- Sensitization of the mesolimbic system.
- Long-term neurotoxicity.

2. Investigational Treatments or off-label Use

Drug	Mechanism	Comments
Bupropion	DA/NA Reuptake Inhibitor	Useful if there are depressive symptoms and mild craving.
Topiramate	Modula GABA y glutamato	It can reduce craving, but with adverse effects.
Modafinil	Mild stimulant, wakefulness promoter	Improves cognition and reduces anhedonia.
Disulfiram	Inhibits DA-beta-hydroxylase	Risk of hypertension; Rigorous monitoring.

Clinical case

Pedro, 40 years old, with chronic cocaine use and ADHD. Bupropion + stimulus control therapy is initiated. Partial improvement. Topiramate is added. After 8 weeks, he reports a significant decrease in craving.

D. Cannabis

There are no specific drugs approved. Options in complex clinical cases:

- **Gabapentin/pregabalin:** for anxiety, post-withdrawal irritability.

- **SSRIs/MAOIs:** if there are depressive symptoms or social phobia.

- **Motivational therapy + groups:** axis of the treatment.

E. Benzodiazepines and Sedatives

Location	Intervention
Chronic use	Tapering with diazepam
Acute poisoning	Consider flumazenil only if there is a life-threatening risk
Post-detox	SSRIs or buspirone if there is residual anxiety

Critical note: Patients with chronic use of poorly prescribed BZDs due to anxiety require delicate management. Abstinence can last for weeks.

6.3.4 Behavioral Addictions (Gambling, Sex, Shopping, Food, Technology)

Type	Possible Medications	Mechanism/ Justification
Gambling addiction	Naltrexona, ISRS	Dopaminergic modulation
Sexual addiction	Naltrexone, SSRIs, antiandrogens in extreme cases	Boost reduction
Compulsive Buying	ISRS, lamotrigina, topiramate	Regulate impulsivity and anxiety
Comida (bingeeating)	Lisdexamfetamine, topiramate	Documented efficacy in certain Profiles

6.3.5 Ethical and Practical Considerations

- Does the patient have a history of drug abuse?
- Is there family or therapeutic support that guarantees supervision?
- What level of insight does the patient have about their addiction?
- Is it a priority to treat addiction or psychiatric comorbidity?

Unlinked pharmacotherapy is an island. Medicine, without listening, is just chemistry.

Conclusion

Medicines, well used, **do not replace the will, but make it possible**. They can support, underpin and accompany, and facilitate. They are the physiology allied to psychotherapy. But if there is no therapeutic process, **the molecule dissolves silently**. Sometimes it's not the medication that saves, but the fact that someone trusts that they can help you (Figure 33).

6.4 Effective Psychological Therapies

Stopping consumption is not the end of the tunnel: it is the moment when one dares to walk in the dark.

6.4.1 Beyond Abstinence

Leaving the substance is just the first crack through which light can enter. Addiction isn't just a habit: it's a symptom of something deeper —trauma, emptiness, unheard needs, distorted thought structures, unintegrated emotions.

Psychological **therapies** do not come to repress behavior, but to **transform the individual's link with his internal and external world**. They are maps to explore pain, tools to sustain it and ways to resignify it.

While the drug silences, the therapy puts words. While consumption dissociates, therapy links. While addiction erases history, psychotherapy rewrites it.

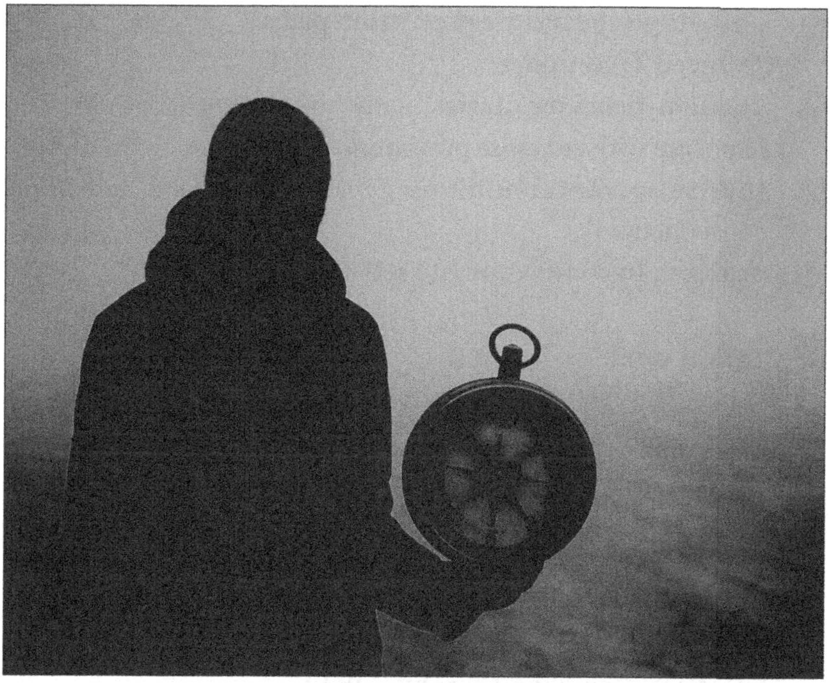

Figure 33. The pharmacological compass. In the fog of uncertainty, a figure holds a compass. It does not point to the north, but to the right time. Instead of geographical coordinates, their marks are human. The needle does not seek direction... Look for the right time. Because in psychiatry, the when is as important as the what.

6.4.2 Cognitive Behavioral Therapy (CBT)

Re-educating the Mind so that it Stops Sabotaging the Soul

Fundamentals

-Addictions are sustained by distorted automatic thoughts, negative beliefs ("I am a failure", "I am not worthy", "I cannot bear this") and reinforced associations between emotion-impulse-behavior.

Therapeutic Objectives

- Identify and question irrational thoughts.
- Understand the emotion-craving-consumption cycle.
- Strengthen decision-making based on reason and not on impulse.

- Design specific relapse prevention plans.

Advanced Techniques

- **Thought-behavior diaries** (daily monitoring).
- **Exposure with response prevention** (desensitization to craving).
- **Inverse operant conditioning** (associating the drug with its real consequences).
- **Training in compassionate self-talk.**

Clinical case

Andrés, 36 years old, executive with cocaine addiction. He believes, "If I show myself weak, they destroy me". CBT allows you to identify this belief learned in your military childhood. Learn that vulnerability is not weakness. One day, in front of her therapist, she allows herself to cry for the first time. He says, "I never thought that talking could calm more than consume".

Dialectical Behavior Therapy (DBT)

When the soul is at war with itself.

Indications:

- Addiction + extreme impulsivity.
- Self-harm, suicide attempts, emotional polarization.
- Borderline personality disorders or history of complex trauma.

Dialectical Foundation:

All healing is born from **the integration of two opposite poles**:

- **Radically accept the present reality.**
- **Actively work to change it.**

Axes of the treatment

Skills training:

1- **Mindfulness:** observe without judging.

2- **Tolerance to discomfort:** resist without harming.

3- **Emotional regulation:** recognizing, naming, modulating.

4- **Interpersonal effectiveness:** asking, saying no, nurturing bonds.

Clinical case

Lucía, 25 years old, alcohol addiction and self-harm. Your DBT includes discomfort tolerance practices when you feel like cutting. The therapist teaches him to immerse his face in ice water: a physiological anchor. He discovers that he can inhabit anguish without destroying himself. He says, "For the first time, I felt that the emotion was not an enemy, just a girl screaming attention".

6.4.3 Eye Movement Desensitization and Reprocessing (EMDR) The Drug as Anesthesia of Trauma

What is EMDR?

- Method created by Francine Shapiro.
- Based on the premise that **unprocessed traumatic experiences are stored as dysfunctional sensory, emotional, and cognitive fragments**.
- EMDR uses bilateral stimulation (eye movements, tapping, alternating sounds) to allow reprocessing of those memories.

In addictions:

- Most addicted people have suffered early relational trauma: neglect, abuse, humiliation, abandonment.
- Consumption is not the disease, but the anesthetic in the face of unbearable memories.

Objectives:

- Deactivate the trauma-desperation-consumption circuit.
- Recover the narrative power of the story.
- Reintegrate dissociated emotions.

Clinical case

Carlos, 39 years old, with heroin addiction. Every time his wife confronts him, he relapses. In EMDR he accesses a childhood scene: locked in a closet as punishment. Reprocess the terror. He understands that his relapse is not due to anger with his wife, but because of an inner child who relives abandonment. Cry. He hugs each other. For the first time, it does not relapse.

6.4.4 Mindfulness and Compassion

Learning to Inhabit the Present without Having to Flee

Fundamentals

- Mindfulness: observing the present with openness, without judgment.
- Gentle recognition of emotion without the need to avoid it.
- Disabling the autopilot that leads to craving.
- Rehabilitation of the bond with the body, breathing, silence.

Internship

- Body scan.
- Conscious breathing.
- Meditation in compassion towards oneself.
- Recovery gratitude journal.

Clinical case

Felipe, 44 years old, methamphetamine addiction. In guided meditation, you learn to observe the urge to consume without acting it out. He discovers an emotion he'd always avoided: loneliness. He says, "The drug made me feel powerful. The silence showed me that I was only hiding from myself".

Therapies as Paths: which One to Choose?

Every patient is unique. The combinations are flexible. Some guides:

Patient Profile	Suggested therapy
Rigid thinking, guilt, distortions	TCC
History of relational trauma, dissociation	EMDR + mindfulness
Impulsivity, unstable emotions	DBT
Search for spirituality, inner calm	Mindfulness + compassion

Therapy is not about imposing a technique, but about finding the right door for each soul.

Conclusion

Addiction is a way of anesthetizing the unbearable. Psychotherapy is the **patient, compassionate, and technical process of learning to feel without destroying oneself, of naming the unnameable, and of connecting what was dissociated**. Each session is not just a treatment: it is an opportunity to be again. Recovery doesn't start when you quit the drug. It begins when you dare to stop running away from yourself (Figure 34).

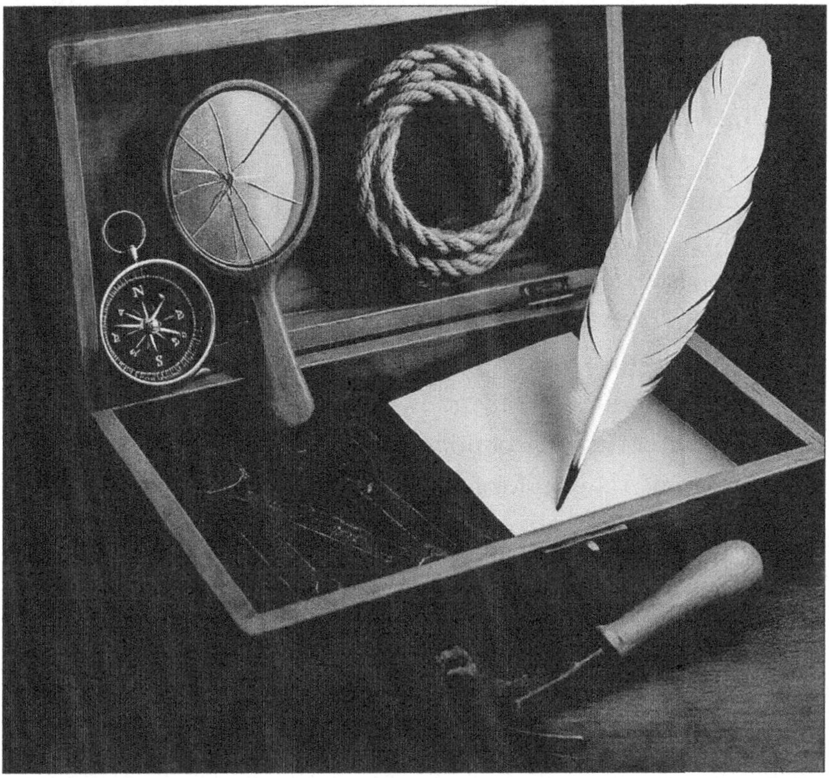

Figure 34. The toolbox of the soul.A wooden box open on a simple surface. Instead of traditional tools, it contains symbols of the therapeutic process: A compass represents mindfulness, which guides without imposing. A cracked mirror in the process of being repaired represents EMDR, which heals broken memories. A rope that joins two ends embodies DBT, where acceptance and change are intertwined. A pen on paper symbolizes CBT, which rewrites beliefs and patterns. This image evokes that each tool, on its own, is not enough. But together, they allow us to rebuild a life.

6.5 The Role of Mutual Aid Groups (NA, AA, AL-ANON)

6.5.1 Listening to Heal: the Power of Peer Sharing

When medicine, psychotherapy and pharmacology have traced the clinical path of recovery, a profoundly human dimension appears: the community. Mutual aid groups not only complement treatment, but also constitute, for millions of people, the true emotional, spiritual and practical anchor that sustains their process of sobriety. This chapter explores in depth what these groups are, how they work, why they transform lives, and how to integrate them into the professional approach.

6.5.2 What Are Mutual Aid Groups?

They are meetings of people who share a common problem (addiction to substances, people, alcohol, gambling...) and meet regularly to share experiences, offer emotional support, develop coping tools and stay sober. They are not led by professionals, but by people in recovery.

The best known are:

- AA–Alcoholics Anonymous.
- NA–Narcotics Anonymous.
- Al-Anon/Alateen–for family and loved ones.
- CODA–Codependents Anonymous.
- OA–Overeaters Anonymous.
- GA–Gamblers Anonymous.

6.5.3 Structure and Key Principles

They are all based on a simple, repeatable and deeply symbolic structure:

- **12 Steps:** A spiritual guide of recognition, surrender, reparation, and action.
- **12 traditions:** the organizational framework that protects the group from hierarchies, money, and egos.

- **Periodic meetings:** open or closed, thematic or spontaneous, face-to-face or virtual.

- **Anonymity:** as a principle of humility, security and collective approach.

- **Sponsorship:** an intimate bond of guidance between more experienced members and newcomers.

6.5.4 The Power of the Shared Word

In these groups, talking is not just catharsis: it is symbolic reparation. To say "my name is Juan and I'm addicted" is to break the silence, to take away the strength of the stigma and to open the possibility of a new narrative. Listening to others tell what one still does not dare to say, but feels on one's skin, produces a resonance that not even the best therapeutic session can achieve.

Shared language is key:

- "Just for today".
- "One day at a time".
- "You are not alone".
- "Your story is not unique, but your recovery is".

6.5.5 Clinical and Emotional Benefits

1- **Reduction of isolation:** feeling part of a group reduces loneliness, a key element of consumption.

2- **Role model and living testimony:** others who are "better off" generate realistic hope.

3- **Sustainment between clinical sessions:** the group contains at times of risk or relapse.

4- **Spirituality without religion:** it allows channeling the need for meaning without dogmas.

5- **Horizontal responsibility:** since there is no medical hierarchy, everyone has a voice and value.

Clinical Cases

Clinical Case 1: Laura, 36 years old, a single mother recovering from cocaine, attends NA and says, "For the first time someone looked at me without pity or judgment. I felt worthy".

Clinical Case 2: Mario, 58 years old, an alcoholic in abstinence for 14 years: "What I could not say to the psychiatrist or to my wife, I said in AA after 3 months. My whole body was shaking. That's where my real healing began".

Clinical Case 3: Alma, 19 years old, the daughter of an addicted father, says: "Al-Anon saved me from becoming his nurse. I learned to love without destroying myself".

Therapeutic Symbolism

A mutual aid group is like a **circle of** fire in the night: whoever approaches finds warmth, whoever moves away gets cold, but the fire is still there, waiting. It is also a **multiple mirror**: each story reflects a part of oneself. It is a **bridge** between the wounded self and the self that wants to live (Figure 35).

Resources & Directories

- www.aa.org
- www.na.org
- www.al-anon.org
- www.coda.org
- In Mexico: www.aa.org.mx, www.na.org.mx
- In Spain: www.al-anon.es, www.naesp.org
- In the United States: state helplines, hospitals that refer to local groups.

6.6 Therapeutic Community Models and Residential Centers

Therapeutic communities (TCs) and residential centers represent one of the deepest and most structured forms of treatment for people with addiction. They are spaces in which daily life, the

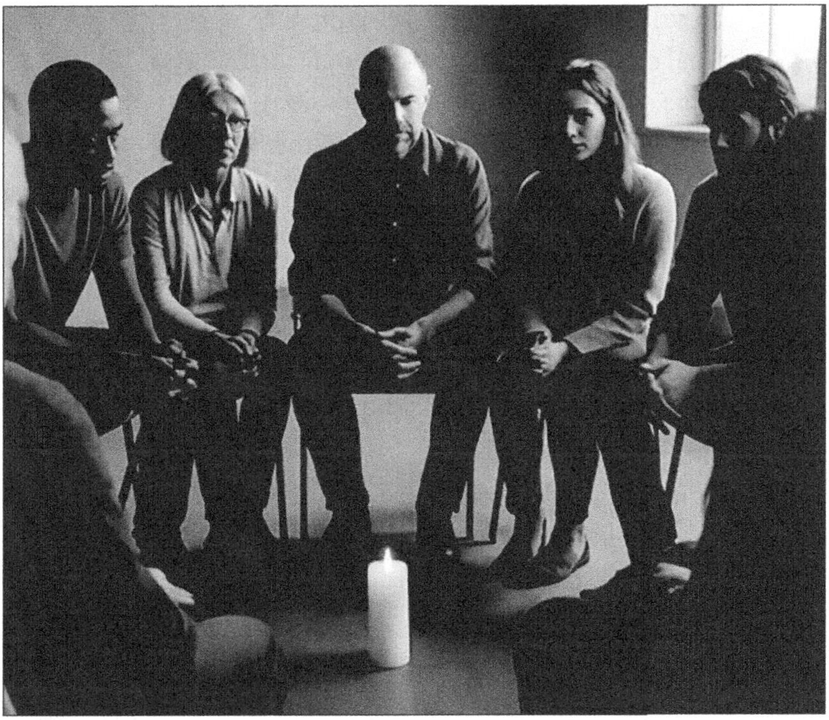

Figure 35. Circle of trust. In a dimly lit room, a group of people from diverse backgrounds sit in a circle; some with their hands clasped, others with attentive looks. In the center, a lit candle glows softly, symbolizing shared hope, presence, and quiet connection. No one is alone. No one is above it. This is the sacred geometry of mutual healing.

bond with others and the shared routine become tools for transformation. Here, addiction is not treated just as a clinical disorder, but as a relational wound that needs a safe, stable, and humane environment to heal.

What is a therapeutic community?

A therapeutic community is more than a treatment center: it is a human ecosystem designed for recovery. Residents are not just "patients", but **active members of a community with responsibilities, rituals, and bonds**. The daily structure includes:

- Group activities for emotional support.
- Shared responsibilities (cooking, cleaning, gardening).

- Clear rules and restorative consequences.
- Clinical supervision and psychological support.
- Retreats, workshops, spirituality or contemplative practices.

Central objective: To re-educate daily life as a vehicle for self-regulation, belonging and existential meaning.

Duration and Phases

Stays in therapeutic communities vary from **3 months to more than 1 year**, depending on the model. Typical phases include:

1- Admission and evaluation

- Establishment of the therapeutic contract.
- Clinical diagnosis and development of objectives.

2- Adaptation and participation

- Integration into community dynamics.
- Activation of social functions: cooperation, listening, limits.

3- Therapeutic deepening

- Intensive individual and group psychotherapy.
- Workshops on grief, trauma, violence, self-esteem, family.

4- Reintegration and exit plan

- Preparation for life outside the center.
- Activation of support networks, employment, housing and monitoring.

Who are they suitable for?

- People with severe or prolonged addictions.
- Failure in outpatient treatments.
- Risk of relapse or harmful family environments.
- Dual disorders (addiction + psychiatric disorders).

The Value of Everyday Life

Eating together, getting up early, tending a vegetable garden or cleaning the bathroom are not simple tasks: they are **rituals**

of reconstruction. Many people in addiction have lived through years of chaos, isolation, or neglect. Shared routine teaches boundaries, caring for each other, loving discipline, and unpunished responsibility.

Clinical case

Roberto, 32, with 10 years of methamphetamine addiction, enters a rural community. It is difficult for him to accept rules. After three months, he begins to take care of the greenhouse. Taking care of plants awakens his emotional memory: "I never took care of it and they never took care of me". A year later, he leaves with a job and a support network. Their greatest achievement: learning to live in a group.

Closed versus Open Residential Facilities

- **Closed:** ideal for patients who are in court, without a family network, or at high risk of relapse. They have continuous supervision.

- **Open:** they allow scheduled outings, family visits, and encourage progressive autonomy.

Models According to Orientation

- **Humanistic approach TC:** they prioritize personal growth, responsible freedom and deep emotional work.

- **Behavioral TCs:** structured, with strict rules and clear behavioral reinforcements.

- **Spiritual CTs:** integrate religious or philosophical elements as part of treatment.

- **Mixed CT scans:** combine several methodologies according to the patient's profile.

Symbolism: "the Inner Monastery"

Entering a therapeutic community is like entering a contemporary monastery. Those who seek to heal from silence, repetition, coexistence and the gaze of the other retreat there. It is not confinement: it is a refuge to reconfigure life (Figure 36).

Global Presence

-**Mexico:** Public centers such as CIJ, private clinics, a wide variety of rural and urban therapeutic communities.

- **Spain:** Proyecto Hombre, lay and religious communities, therapeutic communities of the public health system.

- **United States:** Therapeutic Communities, Sober Living Houses, Halfway Houses, integrated programs with mental health.

Clinical Testimonials

"I didn't come here to be cured. I came to learn how to live again".

"The silence of the mountain and the voice of my companions brought me back to myself".

6.7 Relapse. Prevention, Coping and Resignification

In the process of recovering from an addiction, relapse is a real and frequent possibility. It should not be seen as a defeat, but as a moment of learning, self-exploration and readjustment of treatment. Just as a sailor can be blown off course by a storm, the patient can also stagger when emotions, memories, social contexts, or impulses overflow.

6.7.1 Neurobiology of Relapse

Addictions leave deep imprints in the brain:

- **Limbic system and emotional memory:** stimuli related to the substance (smells, places, people) can activate pleasant memories associated with consumption.

- **Weakened prefrontal cortex:** affects decision-making and self-control, even months or years after you have stopped using.

- **Dopamine and reinforcement system:** The brain still remembers that consumption was a quick form of gratification.

Relapse is a neurobiological expression of desire, not a moral failing.

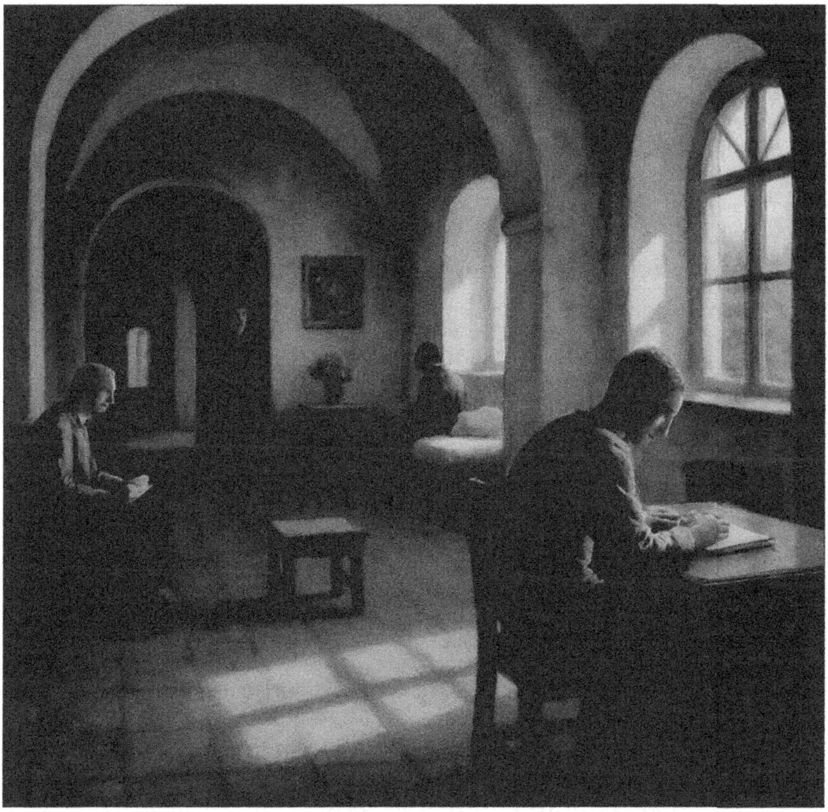

Figure 36. "The interior monastery. A silent path leads to a modest house surrounded by nature. There are no closed doors, but windows open to the landscape. Inside, human figures perform everyday tasks: one sweeps, another waters plants, another writes in a notebook. It is not about confinement, but about retirement. This image symbolizes the therapeutic community as a refuge, where simple, shared life becomes medicine for the wounded soul.

6.7.2 Factors that Precipitate Relapse

1- Emotional: sadness, anxiety, euphoria, frustration, loneliness.

2- Environmental: contact with friends who consume, visits to places of consumption.

3- Cognitive: thoughts such as "just once", "I'm already in control of it", "I deserve it".

4- Physiological: insomnia, hunger, physical pain or stress.

5- Relational: family arguments, love breakups, work conflicts.

Relapse often begins days or weeks before use with subtle signs of vulnerability.

6.7.3 Relapse Prevention: Tools and Strategies

1- Identification of personalized risk factors

- Map of early warning signs.

2- Exposure techniques and desire management

- Exercise "surfing the wave of craving": accepting urgency without giving in.

3- Emergency plan

- Who to call? Where to go? What to do in the first 30 minutes?

4- Social skills training

- Say no firmly, face peer pressure, break previous routines.

5- Daily emotional record

- Tools such as journaling or self-registration APS to recognize patterns.

6- Mindfulness and emotional regulation

- Recognize without judging. Breathe, stop, choose.

6.7.4 Coping and Resignification after a Relapse

Relapse does not cancel progress, quite the opposite:

- It allows you to review what worked and what didn't.
- It gives the opportunity to reinforce the treatment.
- It humanizes the process: it makes it real, imperfect and possible.

Some useful phrases in therapy:

- "What got you there?"
- "What did you learn that you didn't know before?"
- "How can you take better care of yourself next time?"
- "What was different this time compared to other relapses?"

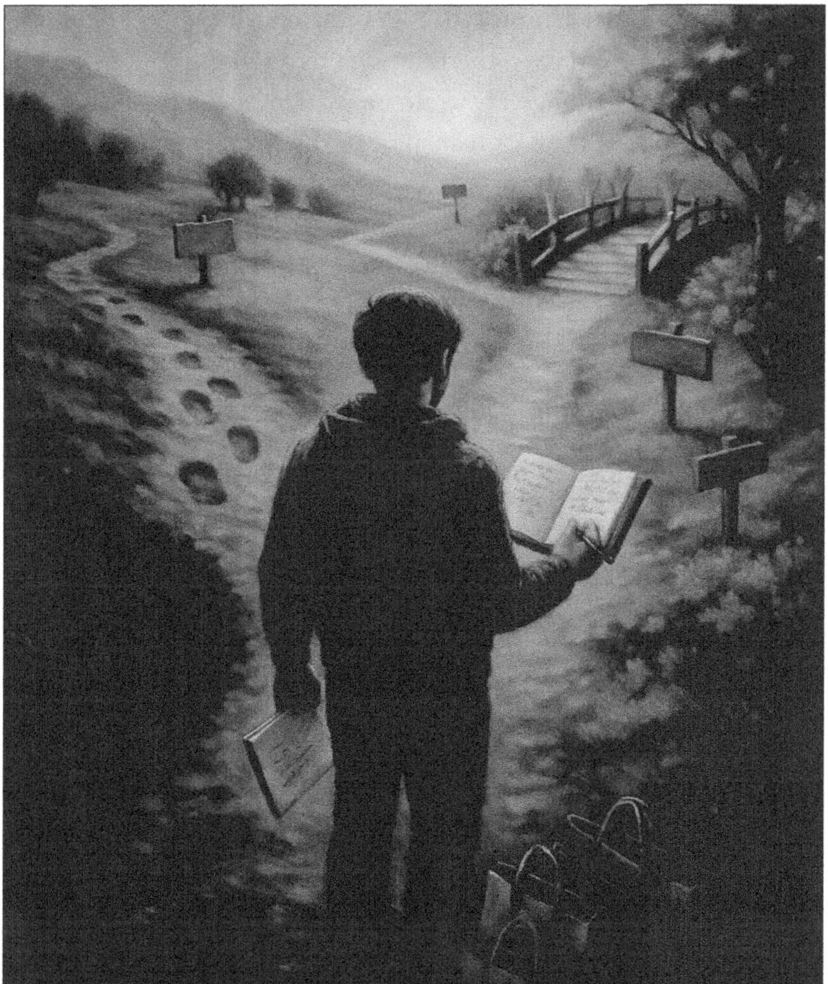

Figure 37. The threshold of relapse. A walker stops at a fork: on the left, a dark, steep path descends into a familiar chasm; On the right, a wooden bridge bathed in the light of dawn, with trees blooming and hands outstretched from a distance. In his hand, a worn notebook: pages crossed out, but still open. This image symbolizes that every relapse also contains the possibility of choosing, learning and continuing the journey with more awareness.

Metaphors and Therapeutic Resignification

- Relapse as a curve in the road, not as a fall into the abyss.
- The garden damaged by a storm, which may bloom again.
- An eclipse: a time of transient darkness, not the loss of the sun (figure 37).

Relapse Help Resources

- Post-relapse intensive therapies in outpatient clinics or residential centers.
- Reinforcement of mutual aid groups (NA, AA, Smart Recovery).
- Tracking apps such as ReSET-O, SoberTool.
- Family circles of guided emotional support.
- Reinforcement sessions with the therapist and immediate support network.

CHAPTER 7
Accompanying a Loved One with Addiction. Family, Partner, Children

7.1 When Love Turns into Pain

Accompanying a loved one with addiction is one of the most challenging experiences that a human being can go through. Parents, partners, siblings, children... Everyone can get caught up in an emotional dance of hope, frustration, fear, anger, and compassion.

Genuine love—that which is born of deep care—can be corrupted by addictive disease, transforming into control, dependence, constant vigilance, extreme sacrifice, or resignation. In this affective distortion, what should heal ends up hurting more.

7.2 The Relational Wound: Loving Someone Who Self-Destructs

When we love someone who compulsively consumes destructive substances or behaviors, we witness a heartbreaking paradox: the person we love seems to be erased in front of our eyes. Their lies, their mood swings, their aggressiveness or their coldness are not simple character traits: they are part of the neuropsychological distortion of addiction.

Many family members then enter a cycle of:

- **Emotional denial:** "It can't be that bad..."

- **Hypervigilance:** checking pockets, looking for traces, interrogating.

- **Constant bailout:** paying debts, avoiding consequences, covering lies.

- **Self-annulment:** to stop living in order to dedicate oneself to the other.

This cycle generates a parallel addiction: **the addiction to trying to save the addict**, in which the family member loses their identity, their peace of mind and their freedom.

Clinical case

The mother of a young man with heroin addiction, she quit her job to "be aware". He sold his car to pay for a rehab center. He pushed away his friends out of shame. When her son relapsed after six months of abstinence, the mother tried to commit suicide.

She was not addicted to any drugs. But she had become addicted to **unconditional hope without limits**. Their pain did not come only from the failure of the other, but from their inability to stop the suffering of others. The treatment, in **her case, involved her also entering therapy**.

7.3 Love that Controls, Love that Annuls Itself

Many times, family members move between two poles:

- **Obsessive control:** wanting to watch everything, deciding for the other, not letting them fall.

- **Personal annulment:** to give in, to keep silent, to justify, to give more.

Both extremes feed the **vicious cycle of codependency**, where love no longer liberates, but enslaves.

"I don't want to lose him, but I'm losing myself".

The true act of love, in these cases, is not to sacrifice oneself indefinitely, but **to set compassionate limits**, to say "enough" from love, not from rejection.

7.4 When Love Transforms: Saving Limits

- **Set clear boundaries:** "I can't give you money if you use it to get high".

- **Get your life back:** don't revolve your entire existence around the addict.

- **Seek support:** personal therapy, groups like Al-Anon, community networks.

- **Accompany without carrying:** be present without substituting the responsibility of the other.

- **Distinguish between the human being and addiction:** continue to see the dignity of the loved one, without denying the seriousness of the problem.

7.5 Symbolism: the Red Thread and the Scissors

Imagine that you are attached to your loved one by a red thread. If you pull it too far, you choke it. If you let go of it completely, it is lost. If you cut it, you bleed. But if you learn to hold it firmly, without strangling, without letting go, the thread can become a guide. That thread is the **love limit**. It is not indifference. It's respect. It is the care of both (Figure 38).

7.6 Resources for Family Members

7.6.1 Mutual Aid Groups:

- Al-Anon: support for family members of alcohol addicts.
- Nar-Anon: relatives of drug users.
- Codependents Anonymous.

7.6.2 Recommended Books:

- Beyond Love: Robin Norwood.
- The addicted self: Craig Nakken.
- Don't drown in the life of the other: Melody Beattie.

7.6.3 Specific Therapies:

- Systemic family therapy.
- Therapist-guided interventions.
- Healthy limits coaching.

In conclusion, accompanying someone in their recovery without destroying themselves is one of the noblest and most difficult tasks. It is not a matter of stopping loving, but of **learning**

to love in a different way, with firmness, clarity, empathy and respect for oneself. Because sometimes, the greatest act of love is **not to save the other, but to save oneself in order to continue loving with dignity**.

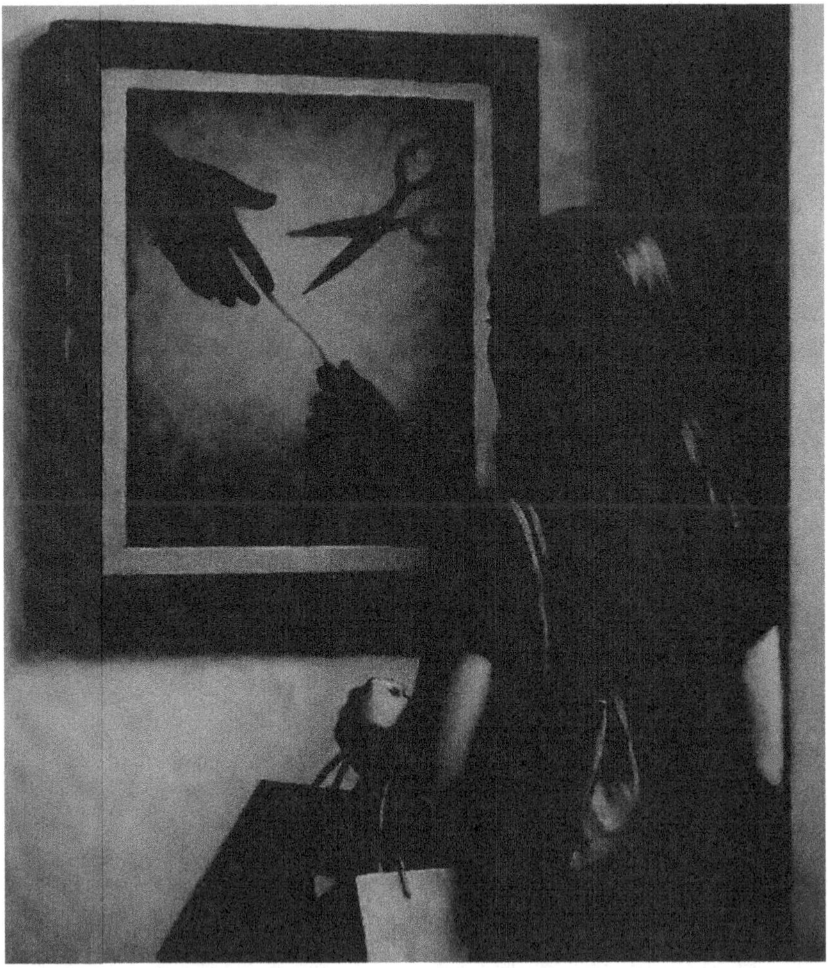

Figure 38. The thread between us. A woman stands motionless, holding a red thread that stretches across a vast emotional distance. At the other extreme, a loved one walks down a gloomy path. She doesn't pull, she doesn't let go: she just holds. All around her, the light of dawn suggests clarity, dignity and the strength to care without losing herself. This image represents the delicate art of loving someone with addiction without sacrificing one's integrity.

7.7 Codependency and Healthy Boundaries

7.7.1 What Is Codependency?

Codependency is a dysfunctional relationship pattern in which one person overinvests in the needs, emotions, and decisions of another, at the expense of their own well-being. Although the term is not listed as a formal diagnosis in the DSM-5, it is widely recognized in the clinical literature, especially in the context of addictions and personality disorders.

It originates in a dynamic where "help" ceases to be healthy to become control, emotional fusion or chronic sacrifice. The codependent not only accompanies the addict: he watches over him, suffers him, justifies him, covers him, and often falls apart when he cannot "save" him.

7.7.2 Neurobiology and Psychodynamics of Codependency

From a neuropsychological perspective, codependency activates reward systems similar to those of addiction. The dopaminergic system is reinforced by moments of "success" or improvement of the other, generating cycles of intermittent reinforcement. On a psychodynamic level, it is linked to early patterns of **insecure attachment**, especially anxious or disorganized styles, where personal validation is obtained through compulsive care of the other.

7.7.3 Clinical Signs of a Codependent Relationship

- Feeling guilty when setting limits.
- Constant need for approval.
- Fear of being abandoned if you do not help the other.
- Denial of one's own discomfort to avoid conflicts.
- Recurring rescue of the loved one (financially, legally, emotionally).
- Idealization of the role of "savior".
- Difficulty making autonomous decisions.

7.7.4 Family and Transgenerational Origins

Many codependent people grew up in environments where love was bestowed in exchange for "being helpful", "not disturbing", or "maintaining harmony". This is common in families with:

- Previous addictions (alcoholic parent).
- Untreated psychiatric disorders.
- Emotionally negligent or chaotic environment.
- Reversed parental roles (the son takes care of the father).

This environment cultivates an emotional hyper-responsibility and an internal sense that one's worth depends on being needed.

7.7.5 The Emotional Toll of Codependency

The codependent family member does not only suffer from the addiction of the other. Also:

- You live with constant anticipatory anxiety.
- Develops insomnia, depression or somatizations.
- Lose friendships, hobbies and autonomy.
- Enters states of hypervigilance (check, review, control).
- You end up emotionally and physically exhausted.

Many times, the codependent also needs treatment, but postpones it because they consider that "the other is worse off".

7.8 Help versus Enable

Help: allow the other to face consequences, provide support without annulling autonomy, encourage the search for help.

Enable: prevent it from hitting rock bottom, justify it to others, pay its debts, cover up relapses, minimize the problem.

Habilitation perpetuates addiction. Genuine help begins when processes are respected, accountability is allowed, and control is relinquished.

7.9 Healthy Limits: How, When, and Why?

A **healthy limit** is not punishment or rejection. It is an act of mutual respect:

- Protects the emotional integrity of the caregiver.
- Define what you are willing to tolerate.
- It puts an end to destructive dynamics without breaking the bond.

Examples:

- "I'm not going to lend you money if you're consuming".
- "I can hear you, but I won't accept insults".
- "I love you, but I can't go with you if you don't seek help".

Consistency is key. A boundary that is imposed and then broken conveys ambiguity and reinforces manipulation.

7.10 Strong and Empathetic Communication

Boundaries should be clearly expressed, without aggression or excessive justification. It requires practicing assertive phrases:

"I support you in your recovery, but I'm not going to sacrifice my health for you".

"I can't control what you do, but I can control how it affects me and what I allow".

"My help is not infinite, but my love does not disappear" (Figure 39).

Clinical case

Mariana and her son Joel (27 years old), addicted to heroin

Mariana has paid for four rehabs, covered debts, lied at work for him, and still has him at home despite robberies and verbal violence. She is exhausted and has hypertensive crises.

His therapist helps him draw a boundary: that Joel can only live there if he agrees to formal treatment. Joel reacts with anger and emotional blackmail. Mariana hesitates, but she holds the limit. Within a month, Joel agrees to enter a detox center.

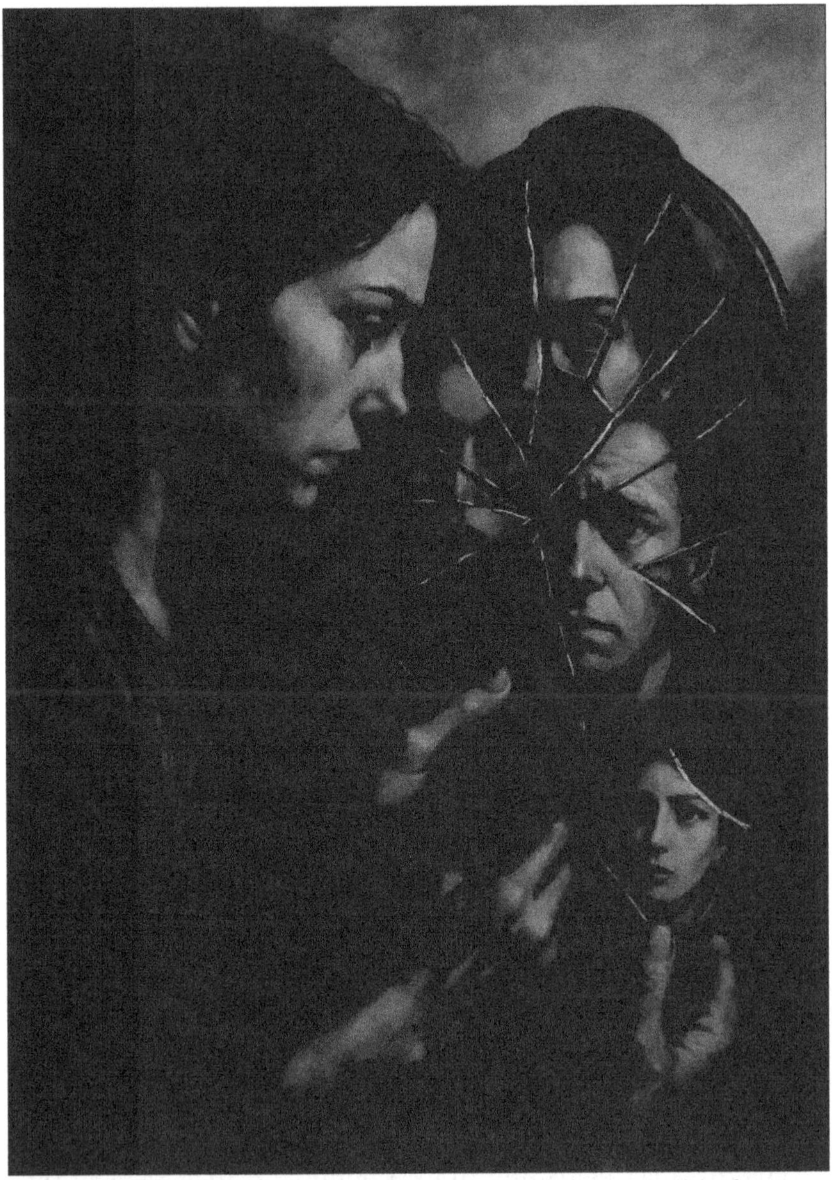

Figure 39. The split mirror. A figure holds a broken mirror. In most of the fragments, the face of another person appears; only in one, his own, scared but still alive. Behind him, the sun rises. This image represents the process of those who have lived turned to the other, and little by little begin to rediscover themselves.

Mariana didn't save him: **she chose to save herself**. And that, paradoxically, opened the way to the recovery of both.

7.11 Healing Paths for the Codependent Family Member

- Individual therapy with a focus on trauma and boundaries.
- Support groups such as Al-Anon and CODA.
- Therapeutic readings:
    1- When to Love Too Much Is to Depend, by Robin Norwood.
    2- Don't be codependent anymore, by Melody Beattie.
- Mindfulness techniques to reconnect with the body and one's own desires.
- External support network: friends, hobbies, spirituality.

7.12 The Role of the Caregiver, Therapist and Support Network

Addiction is not a disease that is suffered alone. Although their experience can be deeply lonely, its impact spills over to the closest ties: family, partner, friends, and health professionals. Understanding the roles these actors play—and how they can help or harm—is essential to achieving a truly comprehensive therapeutic approach.

7.12.1 The Caregiver: between Love, Exhaustion and Hope

The **main caregiver** is usually a non-professional figure: a father, mother, partner or even an adult child who assumes the weight of daily accompaniment. Their presence can be a key protective factor, but also a source of suffering if it becomes a silent slaughter pattern.

Positive Caregiver Roles:

- Provide **emotional stability** and containment during crises.
- Facilitate **access to treatment** and therapeutic follow-up.

- Stimulate **motivation to change** without falling into demands or reproaches.

- Be a **model of emotional regulation** and self-care.

Common Risks:

- **Codependency:** sacrificing one's own life to save the other.

- **Hypercontrol:** supervising each step of the addict, preventing their autonomy.

- **Chronic Guilt:** feeling that your love has not been enough to prevent relapse.

- **Denial of Burnout:** neglecting your own physical and mental health.

"My life revolved around whether he used it or not. I stopped recognizing myself. Then I understood that accompanying is not the same as carrying him". Testimony of a wife.

7.12.2 The Therapist: Professional Guide and Compassionate Mirror

The therapist who treats addictions faces a complex clinical and ethical challenge. It is not enough to understand the diagnoses; it must generate a therapeutic alliance without falling into condescension, frustration or salvationism.

Keys to an Effective Therapeutic Framework:

- **Unjustified validation:** understanding pain without excusing the behavior.

- **Active** and non-confrontational listening, promoting patient autonomy.

- Integrate **eclectic and personalized approaches**: CBT, EMDR, DBT, motivational interviewing, among others.

- **Networking:** Include the patient's environment when possible and clinically appropriate.

The difference between "treating an addiction" and "treating a person with an addiction" lies in looking beyond the substance.

7.12.3 The Support Network: Invisible but Vital Support

The concept of a "support network" encompasses everything from a **group of conscious friends**, to community associations, parishes, AA/AN organizations, and even virtual spaces. Their existence can make the difference between relapse and support.

Elements of a Healthy Support Network:

- **Diversity:** not everything should fall on a single bond.
- **Horizontality:** relationships where aid circulates, it is not imposed.
- **Realistic availability:** being present without cancelling yourself.
- **Ability to confront with respect:** saying what is uncomfortable without harming.

The support network does not replace the therapist or caregiver, but it expands the field of emotional resonance, reduces isolation and strengthens the patient's motivation.

Clinical case

A 34-year-old male patient, with cocaine addiction, began outpatient treatment after an overdose. His partner accompanied him at first, but he was emotionally absent. The mother, codependent, justified each relapse. The therapist created an intervention plan:

- Set up family sessions to set healthy boundaries.
- Referred the mother to a support group for family members of addicts.
- Suggestion of assistance to the NA for the patient and psychiatric follow-up.

Result: At 4 months, the patient continued abstinent. The mother had decreased her overprotective behavior. The couple resumed communication. The net functioned like a fabric that held without entanglement.

In conclusion, accompanying someone in their addiction process is no small task. It involves patience, boundaries, empathy, clinical and human resources. But above all, it implies **recognizing that no one is saved alone**, not even the savior (Figure 40).

7.13 Children and Adolescents with Addicted Parents

7.13.1 When Home Becomes Unpredictable

Children of parents with addiction are not only "witnesses" to the problem: they are direct victims of an unpredictable, emotionally inconsistent, and often traumatic environment. Although they are often the great invisibles of the system, the traces left by addiction in their childhood can last into adulthood, affecting bonds, mental health and identity development.

This chapter explores in depth the emotional, neurological, and behavioral impact on children growing up in homes with active addiction, as well as clinical and community strategies to protect, repair, and help them flourish.

7.13.2 Neurobiology of Childhood Trauma

During childhood, the nervous system is in formation. Chronic exposure to stress – yelling, neglect, abuse, abandonment, violence associated with consumption – activates the hypothalamic-pituitary-adrenal axis, generating:

- Hypervigilance (inhibited prefrontal cortex, hyperactivated amygdala).
- Alteration in reward circuits and emotional regulation.
- Increased risk of developing ADHD, conduct disorder, anxiety, or depression.
- Increased likelihood of consumption in adolescence.

"A child who lives with an unpredictable adult learns to anticipate danger in every shadow. He does not rest, he does not trust, and many times, he does not speak either".

7.13.3 Family Dynamics and Types of Child Response

Each child responds differently to dysfunction. Some rebel, others become invisible. Everyone adapts.

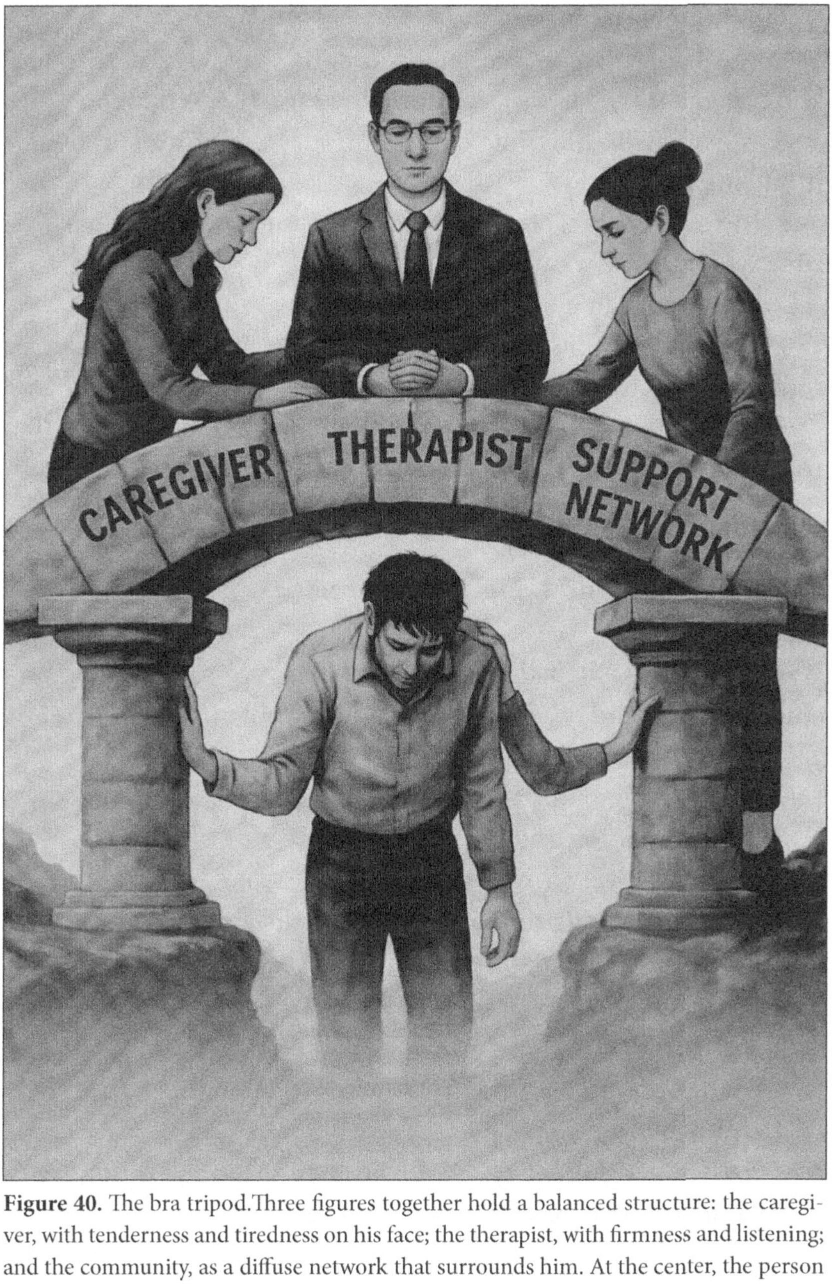

Figure 40. The bra tripod.Three figures together hold a balanced structure: the caregiver, with tenderness and tiredness on his face; the therapist, with firmness and listening; and the community, as a diffuse network that surrounds him. At the center, the person in recovery is kept standing, not by a single person, but by the collective fabric that does not let him fall.

Common types of response:

- The hypermature (parentalized child): takes care of the sibling, manages the house, comforts the intoxicated parent.

- The one who hides: he closes himself in the room, in books, in the internal world.

- The challenger: acts, challenges, gets into trouble to make visible what no one wants to see.

- The comedian: uses humor as a shield against anguish.

- The rescuer: he feels guilty, he tries to "save" the father or mother from childhood.

Each one creates a protective role, but in the long term that role becomes an armor that prevents them from growing authentically.

7.13.4 Short and Long-term Sequelae

In childhood:

- Difficulties in trusting adults.
- Attention and emotional regulation problems.
- Nightmares, separation anxiety.
- Feelings of guilt or family shame.
- Overadaptation and perfectionism.

In adolescence:

- Risk behaviors (drugs, careless sex, self-harm).
- Depression, suicidal ideation.
- Eating disorders.
- Distrust of authority.
- High dropout rates or academic overdemand.

In adulthood:

- Cycle repetition (couples with addictions, self-consumption).
- Codependency, inability to set limits.
- Complex post-traumatic stress disorder.
- Constant search for approval or social isolation.

Clinical case

A 14 years old female patient living with her mother, who is addicted to alcohol. His father is absent. At school she is bright, orderly, "exemplary", but her teacher notices that she gets anxious when there are changes in routine. One day he cries inconsolably when he forgets a task.

In therapy, she says that she fears that her mother "will die asleep" if she is not there. He confesses that he wakes up every night to "see if he breathes".

Her therapist helps her build a narrative where she is not responsible for her mother's health. Internal security, external networks work and the intervention of the social system is activated.

7.13.5 Therapeutic and Community Approach

Stage 1: Security

- Contact with child protective services if there is negligence or risk.
- Include a trusted adult from the immediate environment (uncle, teacher, grandmother).
- Medical and emotional supervision of the child.

Stage 2: Validation and listening

- Create spaces for non-verbal expression (drawing, play, art).
- Avoid judging the parent. Do not encourage blind loyalty or contempt.
- Use metaphors: "your dad has a disease that affects how he acts, not who you are".

Stage 3: Identity and resource building

- Reinforce self-esteem not based on roles (not for caring, but for being).
- Support group for children of alcoholics (such as Alateen).
- Emotional education and regulation of the body (breathing, yoga, child mindfulness).

7.13.6 Keys to Resilience

- A single available, reliable, and emotionally present adult can change a child's destiny.
- Protection is not always about taking the child out: it is about giving them internal tools to survive the environment while they are transforming.
- Children in homes with addiction can leave wounds... but also seeds of empathy, strength and emotional wisdom if accompanied well (figure 41).

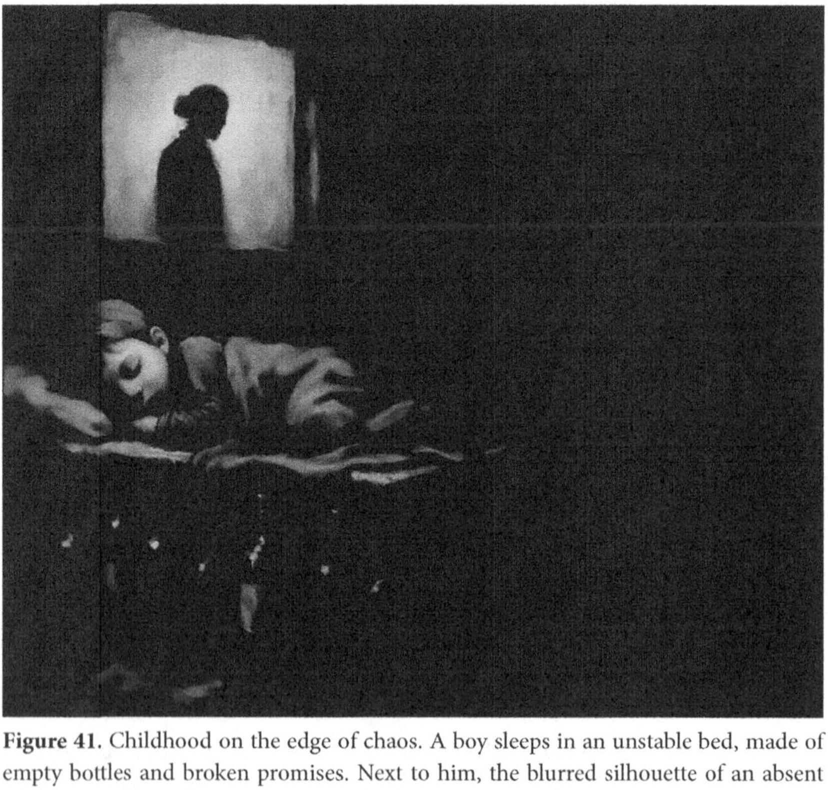

Figure 41. Childhood on the edge of chaos. A boy sleeps in an unstable bed, made of empty bottles and broken promises. Next to him, the blurred silhouette of an absent adult. But through the window a ray of light enters: the firm figure of a teacher, a grandmother, a therapist. All is not lost. Sometimes, a single present bond is enough to sustain the soul.

7.14 Community, Legal, and Emergency Resources

7.14.1 When Everything Overflows

Accompanying a person with addiction can be like living in storms: there are moments of calm and others of absolute chaos. When the physical or mental health of the loved one deteriorates, when there is a risk of suicide, aggression, overdose or total abandonment of reality, action is required. Not from the impulse, but from a plan. This chapter is that compass in the middle of the fog.

7.14.2 Immediate Emergency Resources

Mexico:

- **Lifeline (800 911 2000):** 24/7 care for mental health crises, suicide or substance use.
- **CRIS (Youth Integration Centers):** free care for drug users.
- **Mental Health Centers (CESAM):** psychiatric evaluations and outpatient treatment.
- **Fray Bernardino Álvarez Psychiatric Hospital (CDMX):** psychiatric emergencies open 24 hours a day.

Spain:

- **112 (Health and psychiatric emergencies).**
- **ANAR Foundation (900 202 010):** help for minors and adolescents.
- **Spiral Institute Foundation:** care for people with addictions and dual disorders.
- **Public Network of Addictions (Madrid, Catalonia, Andalusia):** free detoxification and rehabilitation programs.

United States:

- **988 Suicide & Crisis Lifeline (formerly the National Suicide Prevention Lifeline).**
- **SAMHSA Helpline (1-800-662-HELP):** Substance abuse and mental health treatment.
- **NAMI (National Alliance on Mental Illness):** Guides for family members, crises, and legal rights.

- **Psychiatric Crisis Centers (Crisis Stabilization Units):** alternative to hospitals for urgent interventions.

Legal Resources and Legal Protection

1- Involuntary hospitalization: In many countries, there are legal frameworks that allow a person at risk to be interned if they meet certain criteria: danger to themselves or others, or severe impairment of judgment.

2- In the United States: Baker Act, 5150 hold.

3- In Spain: involuntary admission by court or medical order.

4- In Mexico: with a psychiatric medical opinion, supervised by health authorities.

5- Family protection order: If there is violence, coercion, or threat, family members can request legal action without the need to file a criminal complaint against the loved one.

7- Conservatorship or temporary guardianship: in serious cases, it is possible to request temporary medical or economic decision-making from the addicted person, to protect them from harm.

Community and Neighborhood Networks

- **Mutual aid groups (Al-Anon, Nar-Anon, CODA):** accompaniment for family and friends.

- **Parishes, neighborhood centers, lay organizations:** many offer counseling, containment spaces, or recovery programs.

- **NGO specialising in addictions:** in all countries there are associations that offer everything from free legal care to temporary shelter.

Digital support tools

- **Virtual psychotherapy:** platforms such as BetterHelp, Online Psychology, Therapy Route.

- **Family self-care apps:** Sanvello, Woebot, AmMind.

- **Moderated online forums and communities:** Reddit (r/addiction, r/AlAnon), Family Recovery Facebook Groups.

- **International directory of help** in Part X of the treaty.

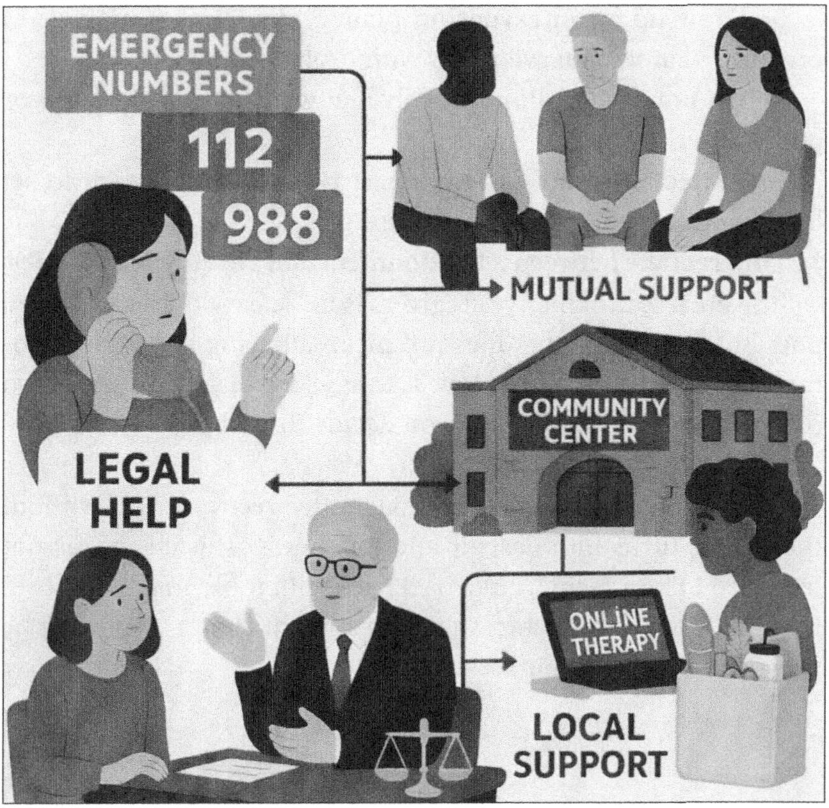

Figure 42. Map of legal and community help. A visual scheme represents the different paths of support for family members of people with addiction: from emergency resources, legal help, free treatment centers, and community networks. Each arm of the map symbolizes a door that can be opened when the family environment becomes unsustainable, a reminder that love needs structures and that compassion can also be institutional.

What to do if my loved one refuses help?

1- Assess the real risk. Are you at risk of dying, committing suicide, or having a psychotic break?

2- Look for allies. Other family members, doctors, therapists, even a justice of the peace.

3- Draw up an intervention plan. Some families manage to organize planned interventions with professional help.

4- Do not face it alone. Involve networks, avoid vengeful or guilty impulses.

5- Protect without destroying. It is not abandonment to set limits: it is mutual respect from pain.

Differentiate between Abandonment and Healthy Boundaries

The great fear of many caregivers is to "leave alone" their loved one. But accompanying does not mean allowing everything. Sometimes the greatest act of love is to say, "I love you, but I can't go on like this. Here I am, when you decide to change".

Shared hope

Access to resources does not guarantee recovery. But without them, love turns into despair and loneliness. This chapter is not intended to be a recipe, but a backpack with tools, maps, and useful numbers. So that when the darkest night comes, you won't be without a flashlight (Figure 42).

CHAPTER 8
Ethical, Legal and Social Aspects

8.1 Criminalization versus Treatment

For centuries, society has oscillated between punishing and understanding those who consume substances. Is it a criminal who uses heroin? Should an alcoholic mother be incarcerated or treated? This chapter explores the thin boundary between crime and disease, between punishment and compassion.

8.2 A Brief History of the Criminalization of Consumption

- **Nineteenth century:** substances such as opium, cocaine and cannabis were legal and sold in pharmacies.

- **Twentieth century:** with the rise of pharmacology and morality movements, a prohibitionist logic was imposed:

1- In the United States, laws such as the Harrison Narcotics Act (1914) and later Nixon's Waron Drugs (1971) led to mass criminalization.

2- In Latin America, the repression of drug trafficking was confused with the repression of the consumer.

3- **Consequently**, millions of people imprisoned for simple possession, especially poor young people and minorities.

8.3 Sick or Delinquents? The Two Models

Punitive Model	Health Model
See the consumer as an offender	He sees him as a patient
It is based on punishment	It is based on treatment

Punitive Model	Health Model
Use jail or fines	Use health, rehabilitation, and prevention centers
Stigmatizes	Accompany and rehumanize

The **punitive** model generates fear, marginalization and recidivism.

The **health model** recognizes the biological, psychological, and social substrate of addiction.

8.4 International Comparisons

United States:

- Country with the highest number of prisoners for drug-related crimes.
- However, programs like the Drug Courts try to redirect treatment instead of prison.

Portugal:

-Decriminalized personal consumption in 2001.
- Result: reduction in deaths from overdose, HIV and recidivism.

Mexico and Latin America:

- The criminal approach predominates.
- Prison overcrowding with scarce therapeutic resources.

Spain:

- Advances in mental health integration, prevention and harm reduction.

8.5 Consequences of Criminalization

- Social: loss of employment, housing, civil rights.
- Psychological: humiliation, prison trauma, increased impulsivity.
- Relatives: children without a father or mother, perpetuation of the cycle of exclusion.

- Epidemiological: more infections of HIV, hepatitis and relapses without treatment.

8.6 Ethics, Humanity, and Reform

- Is it ethical to punish someone for having a disease that harms their own body?

- Addiction **is not a free decision** in its advanced phase: there is compulsion, deterioration and suffering.

- Untreated punishment **does not prevent** or **cure**, it only deepens the pain.

8.7 Real alternatives: Treatment Instead of Prison

- Drug courts: evaluate and redirect to treatment.

- Mandatory treatment centers: under judicial supervision.

- Harm reduction programs: clean syringes, naloxone, supervised consumption rooms.

- Community education: to reduce stigma and promote accompaniment.

8.8 The New Paradigm: Health as Justice

A fair system is not the one that punishes the most, but the one that **heals the best**. The paradigm shift must be global:

- View addiction as a public health problem, not a crime.

- Offer accessible, dignified and culturally relevant treatment.

- Reinsert instead of exclude.

Clinical Testimony

"I was imprisoned three times for possession. They never offered me help. In prison I consumed more. It was only when a psychologist looked me in the eye and told me that I was not a delinquent, that I began to change" (Mario, 42 years old, Mexico).

Conclusions

- Criminalization has not solved the problem: it has aggravated it.

- Addiction should be treated, not punished.

- True justice is built with humanity, science and prevention (Figure 43).

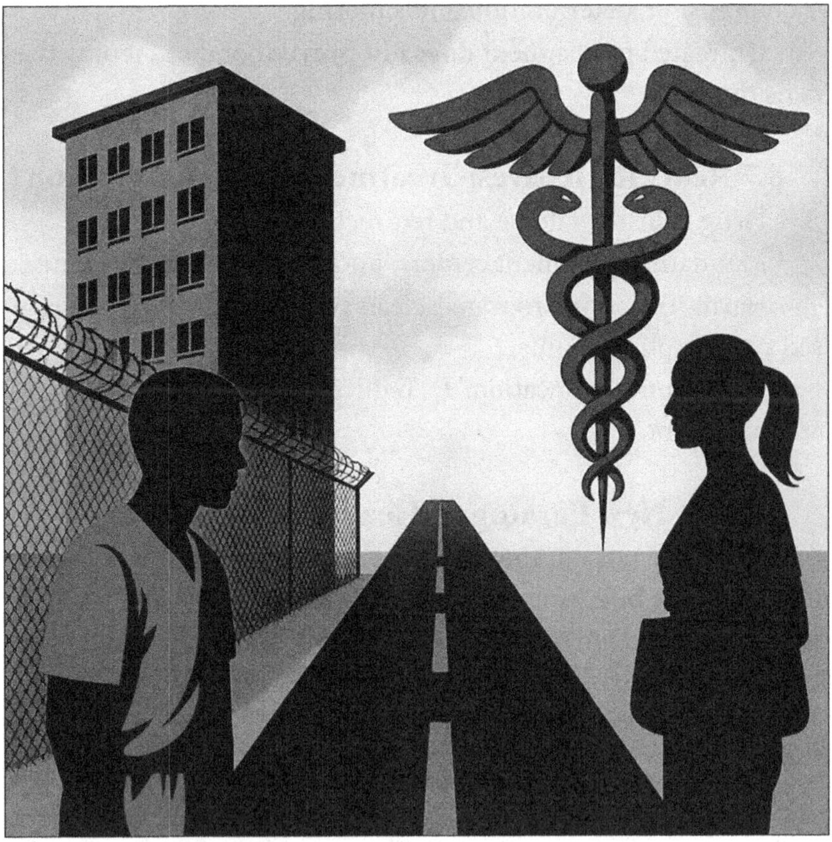

Figure 43. Between bars and hope. Two paths open up before a solitary figure: one leads to a dark cell, the other to a lighted clinic. This crossroads represents the ethical and social decision to treat or punish those living with addiction. On the horizon, compassion appears as the bridge that can unite justice and health.

CHAPTER 9
Addiction in the Homeless Population. When Marginality, Trauma, and Addiction are Intertwined

9.1 A Silenced Reality: Statistics and Forgotten Faces

The homeless population represents one of the crudest expressions of social exclusion. Although official censuses often underestimate their magnitude, it is estimated that:

- In **the United States**, more than **580,000 people** are experiencing homelessness, and about 38% report active substance use.

- In **Mexico**, it is estimated that more than **20,000 people** live on the streets of large cities such as Mexico City, Guadalajara or Tijuana, with a high consumption of inhalants, alcohol and crystal.

- In **Spain**, around **33,000** people live in conditions of homelessness, many trapped in a cycle of addiction and social exclusion.

Behind these figures are stories marked by abandonment, violence, mental illness and lack of opportunities.

9.2 The Street-Addiction-Street Cycle: a Spiral of Exclusion

The relationship between the street and addiction is not unidirectional. There are those who **come to the street because of their addiction**, but there are also those who **develop addiction as a response to the street**. This vicious circle can be summarized as follows:

1- **Social or family displacement** → loss of housing

2- **Extreme conditions**: cold, hunger, violence, → use of drugs as emotional anesthesia

3- **Criminalization** and stigmatization → barriers to access to services

4- **Further** physical and mental deterioration and → perpetuation of homelessness

The use of substances fulfills, in many cases, a psychological **survival function** in the face of emptiness, fear or pain.

9.3 Low-cost, High-harm Drugs

On the street, access to drugs is often mediated by availability, price, and quick effect. Some common substances include:

- **Inhalants (tinker, active, gasoline)**: cheap, accessible, but highly neurotoxic.

- **Crystal (methamphetamine)**: used for its energizing and anorectic effect.

- **Adulterated or recycled alcohol** (called "thirty-three", "chirris"): frequent cause of poisoning and death.

- **Heroin and fentanyl:** in countries such as the United States, they have replaced prescription opioids, with very high overdose mortality.

Often, these substances are consumed **in lethal combination**, without medical knowledge or supervision, aggravating physical and mental deterioration.

9.4 Barriers to Access to Treatment

People in street situations face **multiple barriers** to receiving comprehensive care:

- Lack of documents or official identification.

- Distrust of institutions due to previous experiences of abuse.

- Stigmatization by health personnel.

- Strict requirements to access shelters or treatment centers (being sober, having relatives, etc.).

Many times, traditional treatment strategies (prolonged hospitalization, formal hospitalization, economic requirements) are impracticable in this context.

9.5 Effective Interventions: between Dignity, Health, and Reality

New strategies have proven to be more effective in working with people on the street and active consumption. Among them:

1. Housing First Model

Provide first decent housing **without preconditions of abstinence**, and then integrate psychological, medical, and social treatment.

2. Mobile Harm Reduction Units

Vans or brigades that offer clean syringes, naloxone, dressings and active listening. Example: Safe Injection Vans in Canada or street mental health programs in Madrid and Los Angeles.

3. Interdisciplinary Community Teams

Psychiatrists, social workers, therapists, and peer advocates who build trust on the street and link to resources progressively.

4. Narrative Therapy and Trauma Approach

It's crucial to work on **complex trauma**, **early abandonment**, **dissociation**, and shame, not just the consumption itself.

Clinical Testimonials

"I don't take drugs to be crazy, I do drugs so I don't commit suicide" (Luis, 43, lives on a bridge in Monterrey).

"Nobody cares about what I have inside. They only see the cardboard I sleep on and the pipe I smoke". (Miriam, 29 years old, homeless in Los Angeles).

These testimonies force us to **look beyond the symptom**, towards the human suffering that is hidden in street addiction.

9.6 Ethical Implications and Recommendations

Working with this population is not only a clinical challenge, but also **an ethical and political responsibility**:

- **Avoid the criminalization** of consumption or the condition of homelessness.

- **Humanize treatment**, based on dignity and not moral judgment.

- **Increase public resources** for shelters with therapeutic accompaniment.

- **Train professionals in trauma**, harm reduction, and intercultural empathy (Figure 44).

For Professionals: Practical Keys

- Don't demand abstinence as a condition of listening.
- Use language without labels ("person in use" instead of "drug addict").
- Bring information material, water, clean clothes: small gestures, great confidence.
- Contact local support networks: shelters, community centers, solidarity groups.

Recommended Resources

- The National Alliance to End Homelessness (United States): www.endhomelessness.org
- Network of Care for the Homeless (Spain).
- Harm Reduction Collectives in Latin America.
- Housing First Europe Hub.
- Documentary The Weight of the Soul (about addiction and the street in Chile).

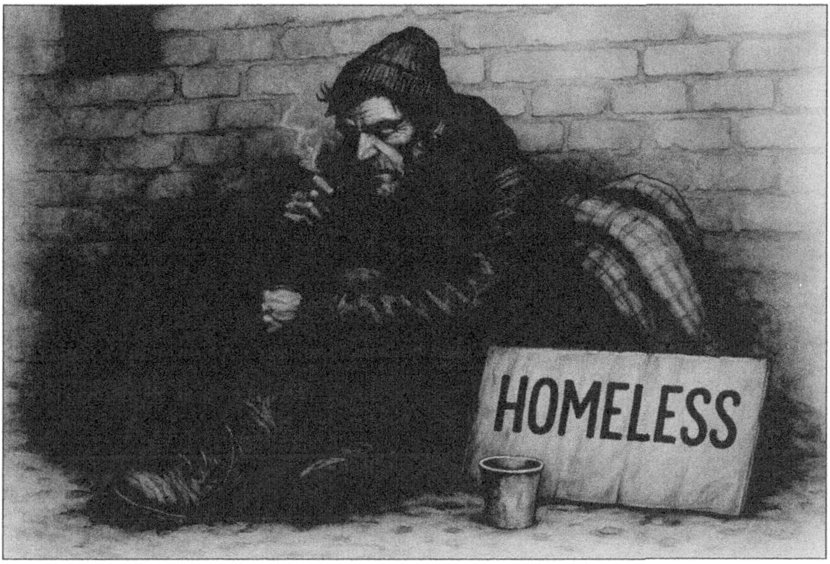

Figure 44. Between cardboard and resistance. A homeless man, covered by worn-out blankets, stands silently next to a wall where aid leaflets hang. The image portrays the intersection between abandonment and hope. Even in marginality, dignity seeks space to sustain itself.

CHAPTER 10
Human Rights, Discrimination and Access to Health. Addiction as a Matter of Justice, Dignity and Equity

10.1 Stigma as a Form of Structural Violence

People with substance use disorders face one of the most persistent and harmful stigmas of our time. This stigma is not only social or moral: it translates into **institutional forms of exclusion**. Addiction is wrongly associated with "moral weakness", "delinquency", or "poor choice", justifying discrimination in schools, workplaces, legal systems, hospitals, and social services.

"We didn't help him because he asked for it". This phrase, in itself, reveals how deeply we have dehumanized the addicted patient.

10.2 Discrimination in Health Systems

Even in hospitals and clinics, where the ethics of care should predominate, people with addiction are often:

- **Underattended**, with doctors who minimize their symptoms.
- **Rejected**, especially in emergencies.
- **Verbally abused**, as if their illness were a deserved punishment.

In many countries, addiction treatment is **not covered by health insurance**, or requires longer bureaucratic processes than other mental disorders. This barrier to access perpetuates inequality and increases avoidable suffering.

10.3 Criminalization, Poverty and Exclusion

The criminal history of many people with addiction **increases social vulnerability**. The criminalization of consumption:

- It prevents them from accessing formal jobs, insurance, or education.
- It limits their ability to obtain housing or social assistance.
- It reproduces a cycle of poverty, consumption, prison and marginalization.

Indigenous peoples, homeless people, migrants and women victims of violence face double or triple discrimination in these contexts.

10.4 Human Rights Approach to Mental Health and Addiction

According to the WHO, the right to health includes:

- Access to appropriate and timely treatments.
- Respect for dignity, autonomy and informed consent.
- Absence of discrimination based on medical condition, race, gender, or social status.

The **United Nations**, through the Committee on Economic, Social and Cultural Rights (ESCR), has urged States to **decriminalize personal consumption**, invest in **evidence-based treatments**, and **repair structural damage** caused by decades of punitive policies.

10.5 Landmark Cases and International Jurisprudence

Several courts have set important precedents:

- **Colombia:** The Constitutional Court determined that denying treatment to people with addiction is a violation of the fundamental right to health.

- **Canada:** the closure of supervised injection centers was considered unconstitutional for putting the lives of users at risk.

- **Mexico:** Recent rulings point to the State's obligation to offer addiction care as part of the right to mental health.

10.6 Practical Recommendations for an Inclusive Approach

For Health Professionals:

- Be trained in harm reduction approach, non-stigmatizing language, and informed consent.

- Integrate care protocols for people with a history of consumption without prejudice or delay.

For Public Systems:

-Guarantee universal addiction care within mental health systems.

- Removing administrative and legal barriers to accessing treatment and social reintegration.

For Legislators:

- Repeal laws that criminalize personal consumption.

- Legislate the recognition of **problematic consumption as a health problem, not a police problem**.

Conclusion: Addiction as an Ethical Frontier of the 21st. century

Fighting discrimination in addictions is not just a medical issue. It is a **battle for justice**, **compassion**, and **equity**. A society that continues to punish those who suffer, perpetuates the pain that it claims to want to heal (figure 45). "No one should lose their human rights because they get sick". Declaration of the Rights of Persons with Mental Disorders, UN.

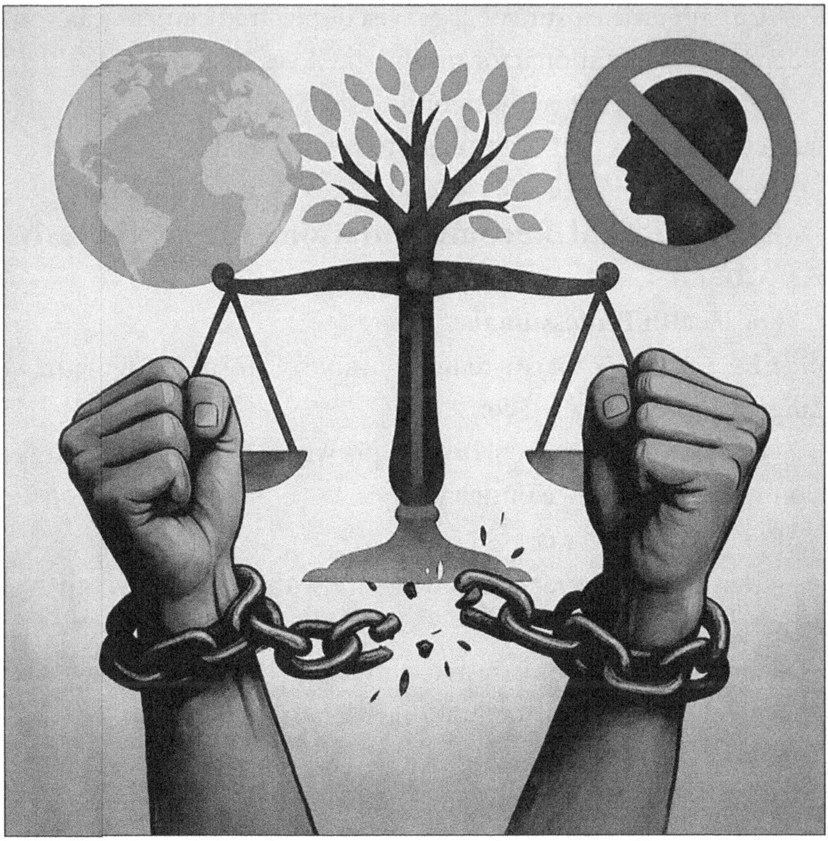

Figure 45. Crossroads of justice and care. A solitary figure stands in the middle of a dark courtroom and an illuminated hospital. On the one hand, the shadow of punishment; on the other, the light of accompaniment. This image represents the ethical dilemma facing our societies: will we continue to penalize suffering or will we open the door to dignity?

CHAPTER 11
School and Community Prevention

Addiction prevention doesn't start in the emergency room, or even the first time a person uses a substance. It begins in classrooms, in parks, in family conversations, and in community spaces where identity, self-care, and psychosocial resilience are formed. Scientific evidence confirms that early, comprehensive and culturally adapted prevention programmes are one of the most effective and cost-effective tools to reduce the incidence of problematic consumption and its long-term consequences.

11.1 Scientific Foundations of Prevention

1. Neurodevelopment and Windows of Vulnerability

During childhood and adolescence, the brain is still in full development, especially the prefrontal cortex responsible for judgment, planning, and impulse control. This neurological immaturity explains why adolescents are more prone to risky behaviors, including early onset of substance use. Positive or adverse psychosocial experiences during this stage shape future trajectories.

2. Protective and Risk Factors

Effective prevention starts with identifying these factors:

- **Risk Factors:** child abuse, neglect, poverty, school failure, family consumption, violence, isolation.

- **Protective Factors:** secure affective bonds, social skills, self-esteem, community participation, healthy adult models.

3. Social Plasticity: the Environment Educates

Addictive behaviors arise not only from a genetic predisposition or trauma, but also from cultural norms, peer pressure, media exposure, and institutional permissiveness. The school and the community act as laboratories for behavioral learning.

11.2 School Prevention: Beyond "Do not Consume"

1. Effective, Evidence-based Programs

Longitudinal studies have shown the effectiveness of programs such as:

- ***Life Skills Training*** **(LST).**
- ***Unplugged*** **(European Program).**
- **Strong Families (Adapted in Latin America).**

These programs don't just focus on substances, but on strengthening:

- Life skills (assertiveness, critical thinking).
- Conflict resolution.
- Emotional regulation.
- Bullying prevention.

2. Teacher Training and Student Participation

Brochures are not enough. Prevention must be transversal in the school curriculum, with training for teachers, spaces for critical dialogue, and creative activities such as theater-forum, multimedia projects, debates and role plays.

3. Emotional Education and Affective Literacy

Deep prevention should teach young people to:

- Name your emotions.
- Manage stress.
- Detect toxic relationships.
- Ask for help without fear of judgment.

11.3 Community Prevention: Networks that Protect

1. Environmental Prevention Models

Instead of holding the individual alone responsible, these models modify the conditions of the environment:

- They restrict access to substances (laws, legal age, schedules).
- They control advertising and normalization of consumption.
- Promote safe and violence-free public spaces.

2. Therapeutic Communities in Prevention

Some neighborhoods create networks of surveillance, mentoring, and support for at-risk adolescents, integrating cultural, sports, and spiritual activities that give a sense of belonging, purpose, and emotional support.

3. Families as Agents of Prevention

Effective community campaigns include mothers, fathers, grandparents, and siblings, giving them tools to set boundaries, spot red flags, and offer unpunished listening.

11.4 The Role of Media and Technology

- Social networks, series, video games and songs influence the representations of pleasure, avoidance and toxic masculinity/femininity.
- Educating in **critical media reading** and building **digital resilience** is crucial.
- Prevention also involves regulating screen time, promoting face-to-face interactions, and detecting signs of early digital addiction.

11.4.1 Obstacles and Challenges

- Stigma: talking about drugs is still associated with shame and guilt.
- Inequity: rural or marginalized communities lack access to quality preventive programs.
- Disarticulation: many programs operate in isolation, with no connection between school, health, and community.

11.4.2 Proposals for Action

Level	Action
Individual	Self-esteem workshops, mentoring, resilience programs.
Familiar	Schools for parents, listening circles, intergenerational mediation.
School	Cross-curricular curricula, partnerships with universities, emotional learning platforms.
Community	Youth centers, community gardens, arts festivals.
Political	Sustained funding, impact assessment, protective legislation.

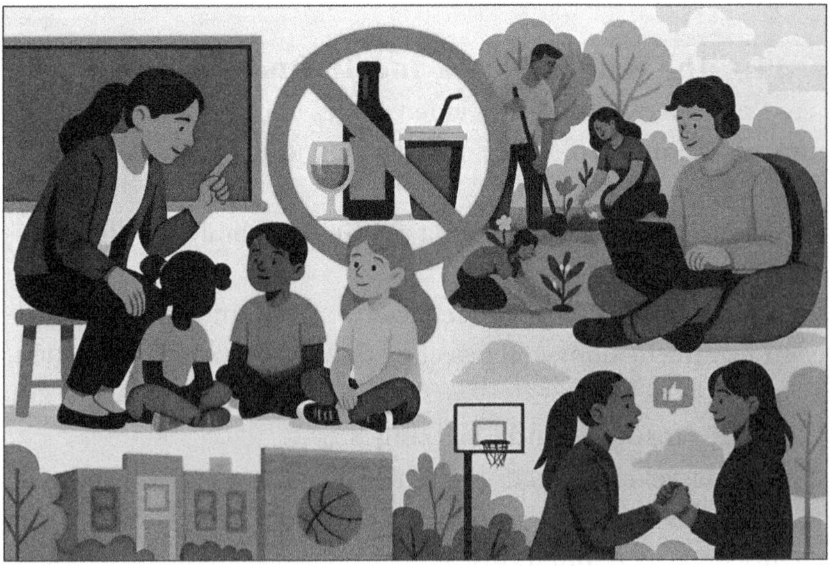

Figure 46. Weaving prevention between school and community. The image shows a symbolic mural where a school, a home, a park, and a community clinic are connected by colored paths and figures of children, families, and educators. It represents how addiction prevention is built on multiple fronts: affection, education, play and health.

In conclusion, prevention is not only avoiding a behavior, but cultivating mental health, belonging, self-love, and critical thinking from childhood. True prevention does not point the finger, but offers the hand. It is a silent sowing whose fruits protect generations (figure 46).

CHAPTER 12
Drugs and Culture: Cinema, Art, Literature and Spirituality. Between Fascination, Tragedy and Transcendental Search

12.1 Cinema: between Glamour, Criticism and Descent

Drugs don't just inhabit public health statistics, clinical manuals, or rehabilitation centers —they also seep heavily into culture, art, and the collective imagination. They are a symbol and a symptom. Inspiration and abyss.

This complexity is reflected in films, novels, songs, paintings and spiritual rituals where consumption is transformed into a mirror of the human condition: pain, rebellion, search for meaning, escape or awakening. Cinema has depicted drug addiction through multiple lenses:

- ***Trainspotting*** **(Danny Boyle):** one of the most iconic, it portrays with rawness, humor and existentialism the life of a group of young heroin addicts in Edinburgh.

- ***Requiem for a Dream*** **(Darren Aronofsky):** it heartbreakingly shows the physical and mental disintegration of several characters trapped in different types of addiction.

- ***Limitless*****:** a distorted vision where a drug enhances intelligence, but with a brutal price: it reflects the desire for superhumanity and its trap.

- ***Blow*****,** ***Scarface*****,** ***The Wolf of Wall Street*****:** they portray not only the use, but the drug economy as an empire of power, excesses and fall.

These works cultivate a double ambiguity: they can serve both as a warning and as an unintentional glorification (figure 47).

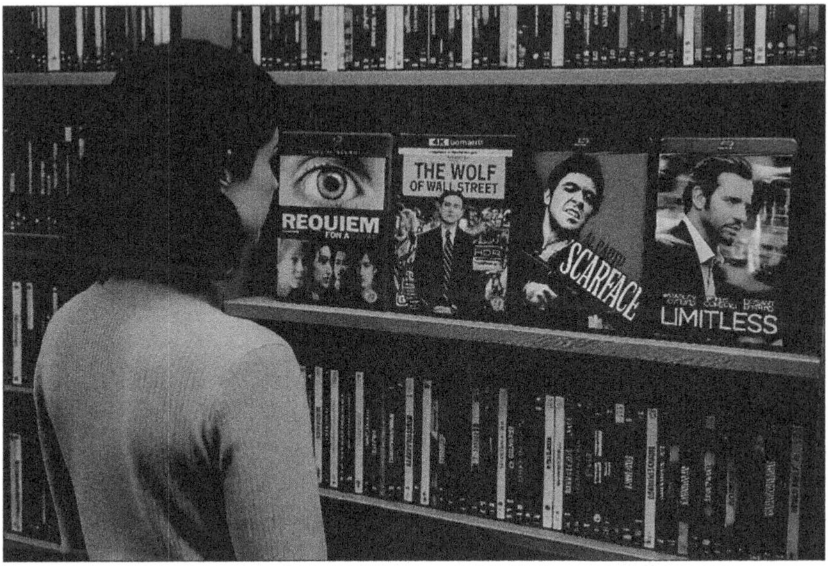

Figure 47. A woman looks intently at a selection of films in physical format that portray the world of drugs, ambition, addiction and personal fall. Notable titles include Requiem for a Dream, The Wolf of Wall Street, Scarface, and Limitless. Each of these cinematic works offers a different perspective on the excesses, emotional deterioration, and delusions of power or escape that accompany substance use. This scene represents how cinema has reflected, critiqued, and dramatized the labyrinths of the altered mind and consumerist society.

12.2 Literature: Cursed Poets and Intoxicated Novels

From Baudelaire and his Artificial Paradises to William S. Burroughs and his Naked Lunch, letters have been a space for exploration with, and through, substances (figure 48).

- **Aldous Huxley** (The Doors of Perception) explored the use of mescaline as a tool for mystical expansion.

- **Hunter S. Thompson** (Fear and Loathing in Las Vegas) satirized the frenzy of consumption as a mirror of cultural decadence.

- **Jack Kerouac, Allen Ginsberg and the Beat Generation** built a counterculture crossed by the hallucinogenic, the poetic and the marginal.

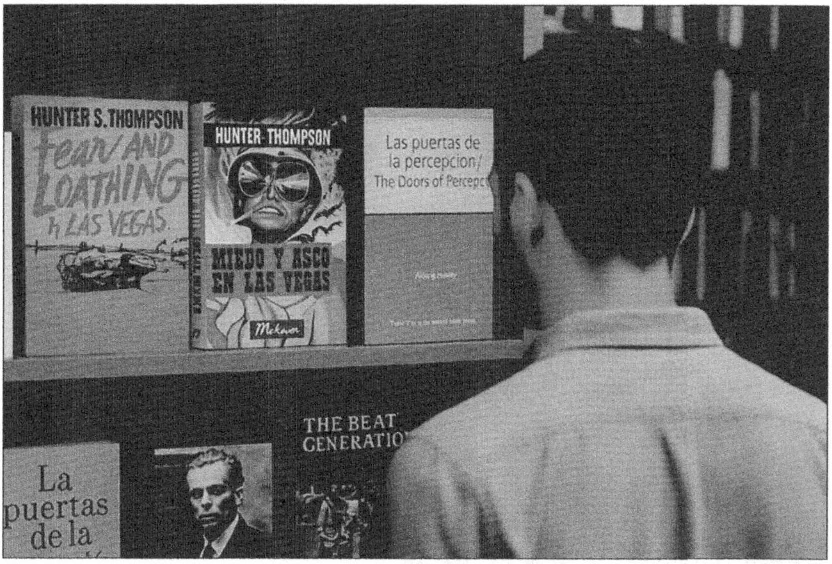

Figure 48. A young man stares absorbed in a shelf of books in a bookstore, where iconic works on drugs, conscience and counterculture stand out. In the foreground, the vibrant covers of Fear and Loathing in Las Vegas, its Spanish edition Fear and Loathing in Las Vegas and The Doors of Perception, by Aldous Huxley, are lined up. A volume on the Beat Generation is also on display, with black and white images by Jack Kerouac and Allen Ginsberg. This scene evokes a literary journey through altered visions, cultural criticism, and spiritual quests.

12.3 Art: Distorted Forms and Transcendental Visions

- **Jean-Michel Basquiat** and **Keith Haring**, consumed by creative energy and self-destruction.
- **Frida Kahlo**, whose work, while not drugged in the modern sense, explored physical pain and the medicated body.
- **Psychedelic Painters of the Sixties and Seventies**, influenced by LSD, ayahuasca or mescaline, sought to represent internal worlds: fractal mandalas, living geometries, archetypal symbols.
- **Outsider Art**, created from insane asylums or in altered states, often shows repetitive, obsessive or symbolic structures linked to extreme psychic experience (figure 49).

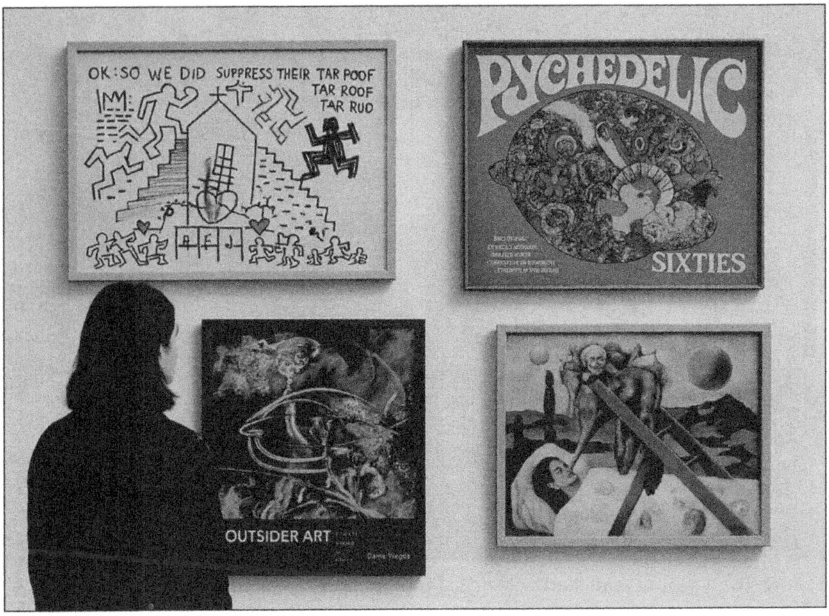

Figure 49. A woman contemplates with attention a series of works in an art gallery, where outsider art, psychedelic and surreal converge. On the wall are exhibited pieces ranging from the energetic and symbolic strokes of Keith Haring, to the visual explosion of psychedelic art of the sixties of the 21st. century. Also noteworthy is the cover of the book Outsider Art, with its visionary and chaotic world, and a dreamlike painting by Frida Kahlo that represents pain, consciousness and the unconscious. The scene evokes the intersection between art, trauma, altered states, and spirituality.

12.4 Music: Euphoria, Loss, and Ritual

Rock, jazz, rap and electronic music have had intimate and ambivalent relationships with drugs (Figure 50):

- **Jimi Hendrix, Janis Joplin, Jim Morrison:** legends as brilliant as they are tragic.
- **Current Rap and Reggaeton:** they reflect everything from street rawness to the celebration of consumption as an identity.
- **Electronic Mantras at Rave Parties:** designed to accompany experiences with ecstasy, ketamine or LSD.
- **Psychedelic Music:** not as a simple accompaniment, but as a sound guide for "inner journeys".

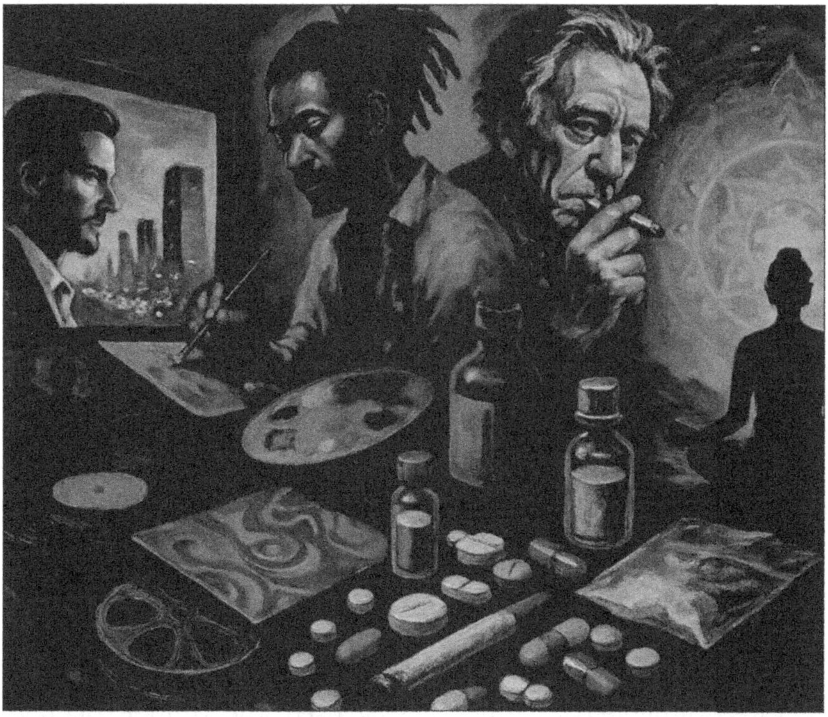

Figure 50. The cultural reflection of drugs. A symbolic painting shows an art gallery where the walls display images from films, books, and indigenous rituals, while various human figures watch with mixed emotions: fascination, sadness, questioning. It represents how art and spirituality portray both the thirst for meaning and the abyss of consumption.

12.5 Spirituality and Ritual Use of Substances

For millennia, certain substances have been used in sacred contexts:

- **Ayahuasca:** in the Amazon, under the guidance of shamans, used for healing, vision and spiritual reconnection.

- **Peyote and psilocybin mushrooms:** in indigenous traditions of Mexico, as a vehicle towards the divine or reconciliation with the lineage.

- **Eleusinian Rites (Classical Greece):** possibly based on entheogenic substances to produce mystical revelations.

Today, many people turn to **ancestral medicine retreats**, combining psychotherapy and master plants in search of deep emotional healing.

12.6 Final Thought: between Symbol and Risk

Culture doesn't simply dictate what to think of drugs: it reveals our internal dilemmas.

- Why are some substances banned and others glorified?
- What does art tell us about our emotional, social, or spiritual shortcomings?
- Can we integrate these cultural visions into treatment, prevention or pedagogy?

Understanding how addiction is culturally represented helps us understand **not only what the addict consumes, but what consumes him inside**.

12.7 Resources to Explore and Understand

- Recommended documentaries: Dosed, The Mind, Explained, How to Change Your Mind.
- Museums with sections of outsider and psychedelic art: Musée de l'Art Brut (Switzerland), Psychedelic Art Center (United States).
- Books: The Medicine of the Soul, by Claudio Naranjo. The Doors of Perception, by Aldous Huxley. Sacred Drugs, by Antonio Escohotado.
- Legal Psychedelic Integration Centers (United States, Netherlands, Costa Rica).
- Ethical discussion forums on entheogens: MAPS.org, ICEERS.org

CHAPTER 13
Medical Aikido Applied to Addiction

13.1 What Is Medical Aikido?

Aikido is a martial art that does not fight the enemy, but embraces him, redirects him, and transforms him. Applied to medicine, it means to stop fighting with addiction to begin to understand it, integrate it and channel its destructive energy into healing. It is not a matter of repressing desire, but of redirecting it with compassion. It is not a struggle against oneself: it is a dance towards inner freedom.

13.2 Who Is this Approach for?

- Those living with addictions, in any of their forms (substances or behaviors).

- To family members, partners, therapists, doctors and caregivers who want to understand without judging.

- To health professionals who are looking for an integrative, symbolic and therapeutic perspective.

- To any human being who has felt the abyss of inner emptiness and wants to inhabit themselves again.

13.3 Medical Aikido Formula for Addiction 2A + 2B + 2C + 2D

Lyrics	Action	Application in Addiction
A	Anticipate + Accept	Recognize the triggers of consumption. Do not deny history
B	Balance + Benevolence	Integrate boundaries with tenderness. Embracing the wounded self
C	Channel + Build	Transforming need into creation, compulsion into structure
D	De-dramatize + Dignify	Get out of the stigma. Redefining the story with compassion

I. ANTICIPATE + ACCEPT

Acknowledging the impulse is not giving up. It is the first step to direct it.

For the person with addiction:

- Recognize when and why the urge to consume appears.
- Do not fight against desire, but observe it and let it pass.
- Accept the story without getting caught up in it.

For the therapist or family member:

- Identify patterns without condemnation: anxiety, loneliness, guilt.
- Prepare safe spaces for when the critical moment arrives.
- Talk before the crisis erupts.

Example:

Miguel, 35, has a craving to drink after work. Instead of blindly resisting, recognize that desire is born out of work stress. She calls her support group, takes 5 minutes to breathe, and channels the energy by going for a walk with music.

II. BALANCING + BENEVOLENCE

Discipline without cruelty. Compassion without permissiveness.

For those who are recovering:

- Create routines with flexibility.
- Not demanding perfection, but commitment.
- Forgive yourself for relapses without idealizing them.

For companions:

- It's not saying "everything is fine", but "here I am with you in the difficult".
- Be firm without being cold. To love without saving.

Example

Laura has not used for three months. One day he has a relapse. Instead of punishing her, her therapist tells her, "You didn't start from scratch. You've learned to come back". Together they reconstruct the prevention plan more clearly.

III. CHANNEL + BUILD

Addiction is a hunger for something deeper. It satisfies the essentials.

For everyone:

- The void that is filled by drugs or behavior can be filled with connection, expression, meaning.
- Writing, dancing, singing, creating, serving, walking.
- Create rituals that replace habits.

Example

Ernesto was addicted to cocaine. In recovery, she discovers pottery as a way to channel her anxiety. Each broken and rebuilt piece reminds him that he too can be remade.

IV. DE-DRAMATIZE + DIGNIFY

You're not a case. You are a sacred story.

- Laughing at the past is not mocking: it is having survived.

- Get out of the stigma: you are not a "drug addict", you are a person on the way.

- Dignify the wound, integrate it into the life story.

Example: Rosa has been sober for years. Instead of hiding her story, she tells it in circles of help. Every time he speaks, someone feels less alone. She has made her wound a bridge.

13.4 Medical Aikido for Family Members and Professionals

1- Breathe before judging.

2- He sees the human being, not the symptom.

3- Celebrate small victories, even if they are not seen.

4- Do not let go of your well-being to support the other: take care of yourself too.

5- Create community: Healing is not solitary.

13.5 The Symbolism of Addiction

Addiction is not just destruction. It is a desperate attempt to relieve unheard pain.

- Where there is compulsion, there is an unexpressed need.
- Where there is relapse, there is a part that still needs comfort.
- Where there is abstinence, there is room to flourish.

Final Metaphor

Addiction is like an overflowing river. It is not stopped by walls, but by redirecting its course. Medical aikido does not ask you to fight against your shadow, but to embrace it, name it, and transform it into light.

13.6 Addiction as a Path to Self-knowledge

To apply medical aikido to addiction is to move with the wave rather than drown in it. It's looking into the pulse of the impulse, taking it by the hand and saying, "I know you came to protect me. But I don't need you like this anymore."

Where before there was shame, let there be compassion. Where there was anescape before, let there be a presence. Where before there was destruction, let there be creation.

CHAPTER 14
A Proposal for Integrative, Symbolic and Resilient Medicine

The approach to addiction has historically been focused on abstinence, pharmacological interventions and conventional psychological treatments. These are essential, but often insufficient. A truly transformative medicine must recognize that addiction impacts physical, mental, emotional, social, and symbolic dimensions of the person. In this chapter, we propose a model that articulates integrative medicine, conscious symbolic use, and resilience development as fundamental pillars of a complete recovery.

14.1 What do We Mean by "Integrative Medicine"?

Definition: An approach that combines the best of conventional medicine (clinical diagnosis, medications, evidence-based therapies) with complementary therapies that have been shown to be safe and effective.

Dimensions Included:

1- Body: nutrition, exercise, sleep, somatic practices.

2- Mental/psychological: cognitive therapy, narrative therapy, mindfulness.

3- Social: support networks, family, community, cultural context.

4- Symbolic and spiritual: rituals, creativity, artistic expression, practices that give meaning.

Objective: To heal not only visible symptoms, but to promote comprehensive and sustainable well-being.

14.2 The Role of the Symbolic

The symbolic as a bridge: Symbols (rituals, narratives, metaphors) allow the person to give meaning to their suffering, find identity beyond addiction, rebuild self-esteem.

Symbolic Examples:

- Initiation rituals, community recognitions, ceremonies to close cycles.

- Use of art, music, dance, writing to externalize the "internal", the traumatic, the desired.

- Personal narratives that are reconstructed: looking at addiction not only as defeat but as part of a learning trajectory.

Integration with therapies: Narrative therapy, art therapy, support groups where symbols and metaphors can be shared.

14.3 Resilience as a Central Axis

Definition: Ability to resist, adapt and grow after having faced adversity.

Protective factors:

- Secure relationship with at least one significant figure.
- Sense of purpose or life project.
- Internal resources (self-esteem, self-control, hope).
- Context that offers opportunities (family, school, community).

How to strengthen it?

1- Mindfulness practices, meditation, conscious breathing.

2- Social support: peers, mentors, recovery groups.

3- Recognition of small achievements: building a sense of progress.

4- Physical restoration: good rest, adequate nutrition, exercise.

14.4 Proposal for an Integrative Intervention Model

I present a treatment scheme that articulates the three pillars: conventional medicine, symbolism and resilience.

Stage	What Happens?	Key Interventions
Initial assessment	Physiological, psychological, social, symbolic diagnosis	Life history, exploration of values, symptoms, existing resources
Medical intervention	Detoxification, pharmacotherapy, medical follow-up	Optional depending on substance and severity
Symbolic therapy	Rehumanizing the experience of addiction	Art therapy, therapeutic narratives, rituals, creative expression
Family Support	Restore link and communication processes	Family therapy, training for family members
Lifestyle and Body Intervention	Nutrition, sleep, exercise, stress management	How-to guides, healthy habits, rest
Resilient development	Strengthen self-esteem, projects, community	Support groups, mentoring, mindfulness, meaningful activities
Maintenance	Relapse prevention, continuous adjustment	Follow-up, plan adaptation, milestone celebrations

14.5 Possible Challenges and how to Deal with Them

- Stigmas of using non-conventional therapies → need for evidence and regulation.

- Financial resources or limited access → low-cost or community accommodations.

- Cultural, family or personal resistance → education, symbolic work of questions of meaning.

- Emotional exhaustion of therapists → support networks for professionals.

14.6 Inspiring Cases

- Integrative Medical Institute, Orange, CA: Combine medication, nutrition, psychological and social support with personalized plans: integrative-med.org
- Takiwasi (Peru): use of traditional Amazonian medicine, rituals, diet, group psychotherapy –a clear example of symbolic and integrative medicine. Wikipedia
- Resilience-based educational or preventive models in university students: how resilience reduces the risk of problematic consumption. Universidad Autónoma de Guadalajara+1

How to apply it in individual practice?

- Design a personalized plan: identify which dimension is weaker (physical, symbolic, social).
- Start with small steps: adopt a daily care practice, a symbolic ritual of your own, build a support network.
- Monitor progress: tangible and subjective goals (how I feel, not just how many times I consume).
- Flexibility and adjustment: what works for one may not work for another.

In conclusion, integrative, symbolic and resilient medicine is not a decorative addition to the treatment of addiction, but its most human foundation. Recovering meaning, strengthening identity, building support networks and cultivating resilience allow not only to overcome dependence, but also to transform it into a door to a life with more fullness, coherence and hope (Figure 51).

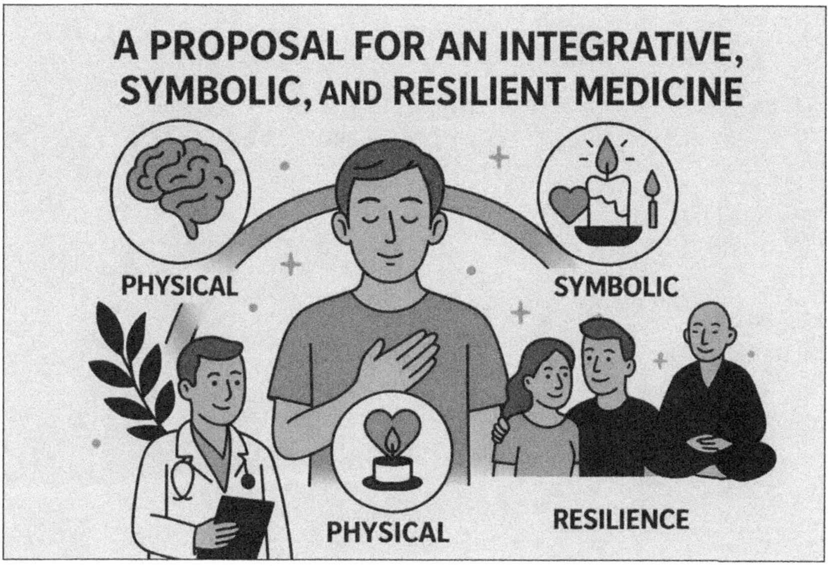

Figure 51. Integrative medicine seeks a balance between the physical, the symbolic and the emotional resilience of the patient. Healing goes beyond the body: a medicine that also takes care of the soul and inner strength.

CHAPTER 15
Resources in Mexico, the United States and Spain

Addiction not only affects the individual, but also their family, social and work environment. Recovery doesn't happen in a vacuum: it requires networking, guidance, and support. This chapter provides a practical map of resources in three key countries—Mexico, the United States, and Spain—with institutions, helplines, therapeutic communities, support groups, and accessible options for those seeking treatment or accompaniment (Figure 52).

15.1 Resources in Mexico

Public institutions

- CIJ (Youth Integration Centers) Outpatient and residential care for people with consumption problems. Present in a large part of the country. www.cij.gob.mx

- CONADIC (National Commission against Addictions) Regulatory framework, prevention campaigns and directories of accredited centers. www.gob.mx/salud/conadic

Therapeutic communities and NGO

- Monte Fénix (CDMX): Private clinic recognized for its comprehensive treatment model.

- Reinserta: NGO that works with adolescents in conflict with the law and addictions in contexts of violence.

- Camino a Casa Foundation: Care for victims of trafficking with associated consumption.

Support groups

- Alcoholics Anonymous (AA Mexico)

- Narcotics Anonymous (NA Mexico)
- Renacer Group: Support for family members.

Educational tools

All About Drugs (educational resource for young people, available online).

15.2 Resources in the United States

Institutions and helplines

- SAMHSA (Substance Abuse and Mental Health Services Administration) Treatment center database and toll-free 24/7. 1-800-662-HELP (4357) www.samhsa.gov
- National Institute on Drug Abuse (NIDA) Research, prevention, resources for parents and educadores.www.drugabuse.gov

Recognized centers

- Hazelden Betty Ford Foundation: Comprehensive recovery approach with scientific evidence.
- Phoenix House: Programs for teens and adults.

Support groups

- AA, NA, Al-Anon, Smart Recovery — Extensive network in English and Spanish.
- Celebrate Recovery: Alternative with a Christian focus.

Digital resources

- Apps as Sober Grid, I Am Sober, Recovery Path
- Podcasts: The Addicted Mind, That Sober Guy, Recovery Elevator

15.3 Resources in Spain

Public institutions

- National Plan on Drugs (Ministry of Health) Coordination of programmes, prevention and attention: www.pnsd.sanidad.gob.es

- Drug Addiction Care Centers (CAD): Free and multidisciplinary care in most of the autonomous communities.

NGO and foundations

- Proyecto Hombre: Recognized therapeutic intervention, with locations in almost all of Spain.
- GIA foundation: Approach from an integrative and psychosocial perspective.
- AESED: Support for families of people with dependency.

Mutual aid groups

- AA, NA, Rehabilitated Alcoholics, Family Groups
- RedUNAD: Network of NGO dedicated to addiction care.

Educational and preventive material

- Guides to the National Plan on Drugs, available in PDF.
- Campaigns such as "#TúDecides" for teenagers.

Common resources accessible from any country

- Alcoholics Anonymous International: www.aa.org
- Narcotics Anonymous International: www.na.org
- Drug Policy Alliance: Focus on harm reduction and social justice.
- YouTube: TED Talks on addictions, educational documentaries.

How to use this chapter?

- As an initial guide if you or a loved one needs help.
- As a resource for therapists seeking referrals or support network.
- As a reference for educational, school or community programs.

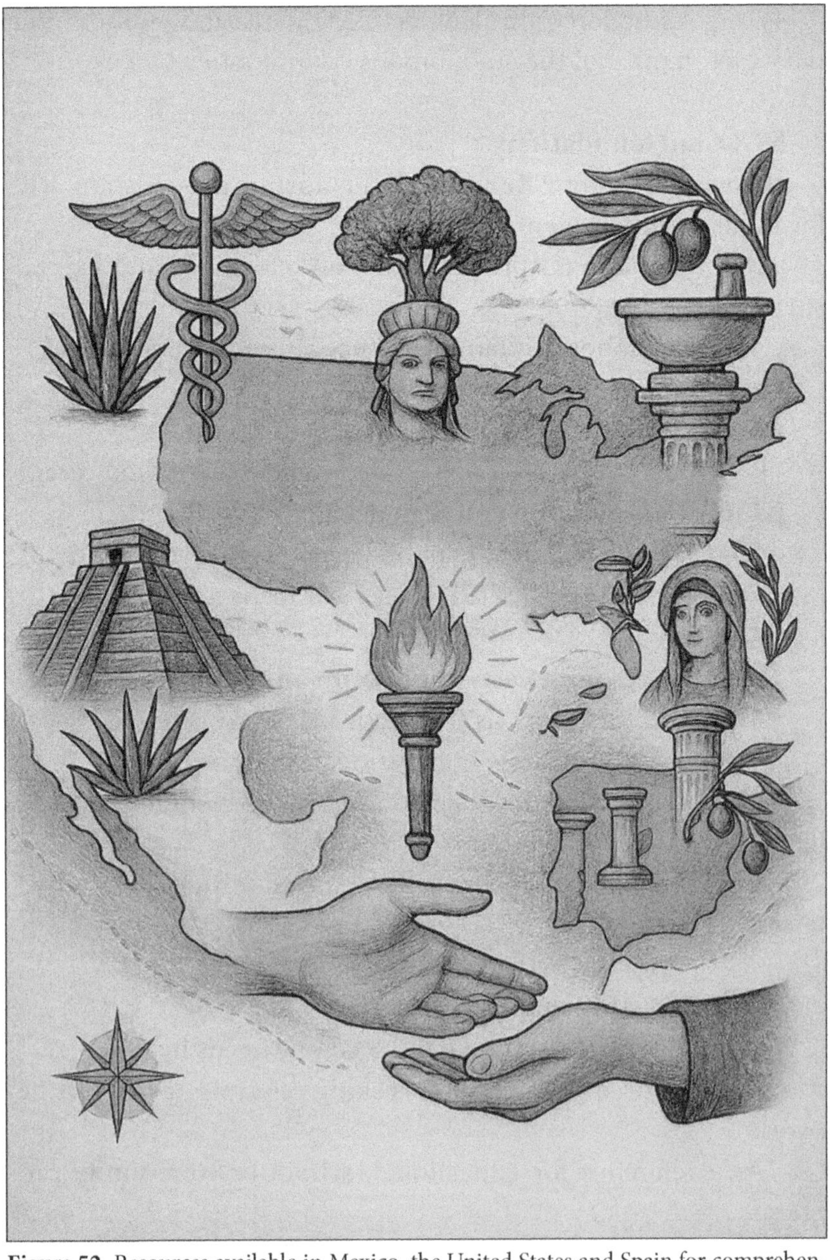

Figure 52. Resources available in Mexico, the United States and Spain for comprehensive addiction care. They integrate medical, emotional, community, and educational support.

CHAPTER 16
Treatment Plans, Clinical Examples, and Integrated Therapeutic Guidelines

16.1 Treating Addiction as a Complex Neurobiological Condition

Addiction is not a moral weakness, it is a disease of the brain that requires strategy, compassion and scientific evidence. The treatment of addictions has evolved radically in recent decades. It is no longer conceived solely from abstinence or behavioral punishment, but from a deep understanding of the **neurobiological**, **emotional**, **social**, and **spiritual** mechanisms that sustain compulsive substance use.

This chapter proposes **a comprehensive and structured clinical approach**, supported by scientific evidence, modern treatment models and examples adapted to different clinical realities.

16.2 What Do We Mean by Comprehensive Treatment?

Effective addiction treatment must simultaneously consider:

- Brain (neurochemistry and pharmacotherapy).
- Mind (thoughts, motivations, psychic defenses).
- Body (physical symptoms, deprivation, vital energy).
- Environment (family, housing, employment, community).
- Spirituality (meaning of life, existential emptiness, values).

Clinical Stages of Treatment

Phase I: Comprehensive Diagnostic Evaluation

- History of use (onset, type of substances, pattern of use, escalation, relapses).

- Detection of psychiatric comorbidities (depression, anxiety, ADHD, psychosis).

- Application of DNP-21–Addiction to identify predominant neurochemical profiles (dopaminergic, serotonergic, glutamatergic, GABAergic, etc.).

- Motivational evaluation according to the model of Prochaska and DiClemente (pre-contemplation, contemplation, preparation, action, maintenance, relapse).

- Assessment of suicide risk, violence or abandonment.

- Exploration of support networks, educational level, work history, meaningful relationships.

Phase II: Medical Detox

- Duration: 5 to 14 days depending on the substance and severity of the withdrawal syndrome.

- Indicated for: alcohol, benzodiazepines, opiates, stimulants.

- Focus: medical stabilization, hydration, management of withdrawal symptoms, psychiatric surveillance, and emotional containment.

- Possible medications:
    - Benzodiazepines (clonazepam, diazepam) for alcohol and sedatives.
    - Buprenorphine or methadone for opioids.
    - Gabapentin for anxiolysis and stabilization.
    - Clonidine to reduce sympathetic hyperactivity.

Phase III: Psychotherapeutic Rehabilitation

- Duration: from 1 to 6 months (outpatient or inpatient).

- Main axes:
    - Individual Psychotherapy: CBT, DBT, EMDR, schema therapy, psychodynamic intervention.
    - Group Psychotherapy: 12-step models, motivational groups, art-therapy, mixed groups.

- Systemic Family Therapy: To Restructure Roles, Set Boundaries, and Heal Bonds.
- Mindfulness and Compassion-based Interventions.
- Occupational Therapy and Reintegration into the Workforce.

Phase IV: Relapse Prevention and Prolonged Follow-Up

- Strategies:
  - Identification of internal and external triggers.
  - Construction of a relapse map.
  - Training in social skills and conflict resolution.
  - Linkage with community groups (NA, Al-Anon, SMART Recovery).
  - Maintenance pharmacotherapy.

16.3 Neurochemical Profiling-Based Pharmacotherapy (DNP-21 Model)

DNP Profile	Predominant neurotransmitters	Guiding Symptoms	Suggested Drugs
Dopaminergic	↑ Dopamine, ↑ Noradrenaline	Pleasure-seeking, impulsivity, euphoria	Bupropion, topiramate, aripiprazole
Serotonergic	↓ Serotonin	Anxiety, compulsion, chronic sadness	Sertraline, fluoxetine, trazodone
Glutamatergic	↑ Glutamate	Agitation, intense craving, flashbacks	Acamprosato, memantina, lamotrigina
GABAergic	↓ GABA	Insomnia, irritability, physical anxiety	Pregabalin, gabapentin, clonazepam (transient)
Endocannabinoid	Affective dysregulation	Anhedonia, irritability, low motivation	N-acetylcysteine, omega-3, psychoeducation

16.4 Clinical Cases

Clinical case 1: Male patient, 34 years old, cocaine and alcohol addiction, without dual diagnosis.

Evaluation:

- Binge pattern of consumption 3 times/week.
- High impulsivity, low introspection.
- Dopaminergic + glutamatergic profile.

Proposed treatment:

- Bupropion 150-300 mg.
- Topiramato 100 mg BID.
- Psychotherapy: CBT + NA groups.
- Mindfulness + physical exercise.
- Family gatherings every 2 weeks.

Clinical case 2: Female patient, 27 years old, prescribed benzodiazepines + panic attack.

Evaluation:

- Hidden consumption of alprazolam.
- High levels of somatic anxiety.
- Serotonergic profile + GABAergic.

Proposed treatment:

- Gradual withdrawal with diazepam.
- Introduction of sertraline 50-100 mg.
- Gabapentin 300-600 mg/day.
- EMDR + DBT psychotherapy.
- Family psychoeducation.

16.5 Clinical Guidelines by Substance (Summary)

Substance	Pharmacotherapy	Key psychotherapy	Considerations
Alcohol	Acamprosato, naltrexona, disulfiram	CBT + duel therapy	Risk of severe withdrawal
Cannabis	No standard medication	Motivational + values therapy	Cultural normalization of consumption
Cocaine	Bupropión, topiramato, disulfiram	CBT + Relapse Prevention	High impulsivity
Opioids	Buprenorphine, Methadone, Naltrexone	Community Support	Requires tight adhesion
Benzodiazepines	Slow withdrawal + stabilization	Therapy for anxiety + trauma	Seizure risk
Methamphetamine	Topiramate, n-acetylcysteine	Intensive intervention	Risk of psychosis and paranoia

In conclusion, there is no single path to recovery, but there are universal principles: treat with dignity, understand the underlying suffering, and design a plan that combines science, humanity, and hope (Figure 53). Addiction is not a final destination: it is a sign that something in the soul and brain is begging to be restructured, listened to, and transformed.

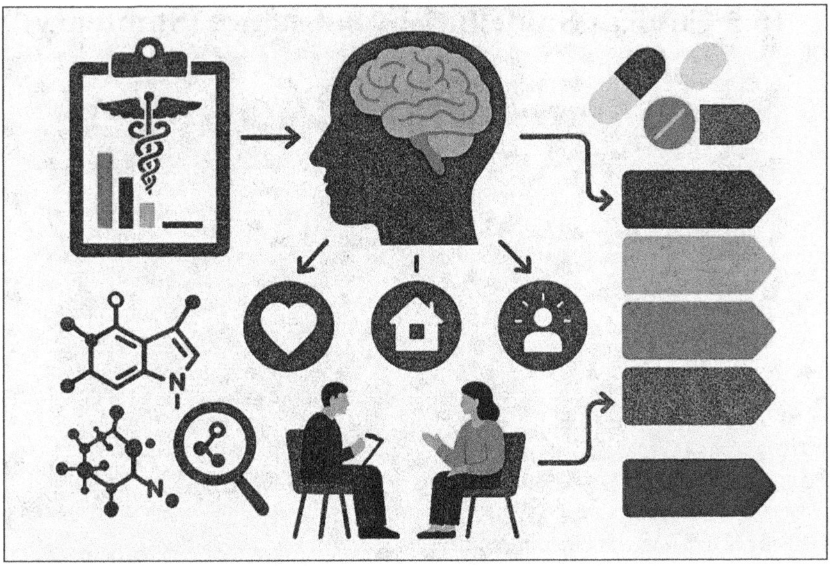

Figure 53. Schematic illustration of the comprehensive treatment of addictions, with emphasis on neurobiological, psychological, social and pharmacological domains, organized by clinical phases and neurochemical profiles. A visual look at modern addiction treatment: from the brain to the social environment, including medication, therapy and community support.

CHAPTER 17
Letters to the Family, Addict, and Therapist

An expressive tool loaded with science, emotion and purpose.

17.1 The Therapeutic Value of Letters

Expressive writing has been studied in psychotherapy as a method to externalize thoughts, regulate emotions and generate personal meaning. In contexts of addiction, a "therapeutic letter" can function as a symbolic bridge between the internal and the external: confronting the unsaid, clarifying intentions, expressing pain and hope.

In group or family therapy, these letters can be read or discussed (when the context allows), facilitating emotional connection, mutual understanding, and candid dialogue (Figure 54).

17.2 Scientific Basis: Why Does It Work?

Studies show that therapeutic writing can reduce symptoms of traumatic stress, depression, and anxiety, by facilitating cognitive restructuring and emotional regulation.

A recent review of writing techniques in psychotherapy states that these interventions promote psychological well-being, self-compassion, and increased personal meaning.

In the case of addictions, the card can be used to externalize the "I that consumes" (the substance or behavior) as something to dialogue with, putting symbolic sanitary distance.

In family therapy, letters allow members to express unexpressed feelings, accumulated pain, or expectations with a lower risk of abrupt emotional escalation.

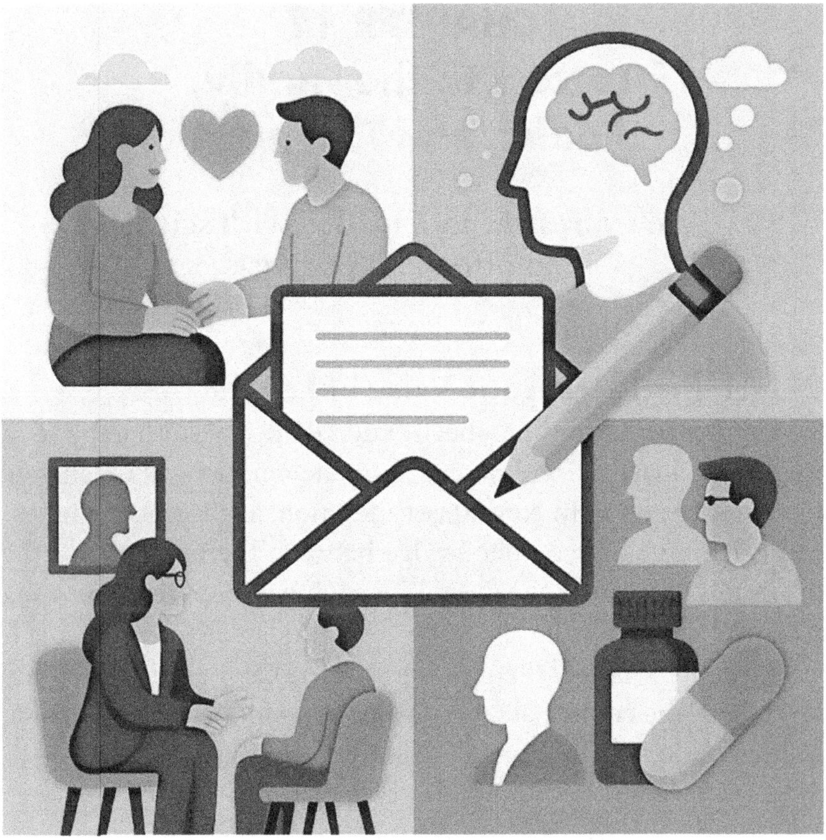

Figure 54. In addiction recovery, the written word becomes a gentle yet powerful guide through pain, hope, and transformation. Writing for yourself, a loved one, or a therapist can unlock deep emotions and start meaningful conversations on the path to healing.

17.3 Suggested Letters: Structure and Narrative Examples

(These are guiding schemes, not rigid formulas)

Letter from the Family Member to the Person with Addiction

Suggested structure:

- Beginning with recognition of affection or bond (what is valued about that person).
- Reflection on what consumption has implied: losses, wounds, visible changes.

- Emotional expression: pain, frustration, hope, fear.

- Clear requests: necessary limits, desired support, intention to accompany.

- Proposal for collaboration and openness to dialogue (without imposing).

- Hopeful closure: reaffirming the desire for mutual recovery.

Example (narrative version, not literal)

"Dear X: I still remember when you laughed loudly... Since you started with ___, I feel like we've drifted apart. It hurts me to see how you changed, how we have lost communication. I want to tell you that I wish your well-being. But I also need to protect myself: I need clear boundaries so I don't feel consumed by your pain. I ask that you commit to attending therapy, maintaining honesty with your process.
I don't ask for it as a punishment, but as a sign that I want to accompany you, respecting my space. Love, you [family]".

Addict's letter to himself/to the substance

Suggested structure:

- Acknowledgment of the pain and harm caused (to oneself and others).

- Reflection on when the relationship with the substance/behavior began.

- What that relationship offered: relief, escape, broken promises.

- Internal demands: honesty, commitment, reparation.

- Promise of concrete steps (therapy, partial/controlled abstinence, seeking support).

- Closing with self-compassion and openness to change.

Mental narrative example (not literal):

"Dear substance, at first you seemed like the friend who soothed my pain. But you took me far: you stole my health, relationships, time. Today I am writing to you to separate. I ask you to let me seek help, not to deceive me anymore. To myself: you deserve to heal. I commit to therapy, exercise, honesty. It won't be easy, but I want to rebuild myself. And even if it hurts, I'm telling you this far".

Letter from patient to therapist (or as a supervisory internal exercise)

Suggested structure:

- What I expect from this therapeutic relationship.
- What fears, resistances or blockages do I feel? (Shame, frustration, relapse).
- What would I like to be understood about my inner world?
- What I commit to do (openness, honesty, intersessional work).
- What will I not tolerate? (Non-constructive critical comments, impositions).
- Closing of the alliance: recognition of the role of the therapist and the client as co-responsible.

Therapeutic value:

- These cards allow the therapist to "see" the client's inner world without interruption.
- In supervision, it can be shared (or not) to dialogue about resistance, transference, blocks.
- In qualitative studies, patients have reported that receiving letters generated "connection, amazement, consolidation of what was worked on in session".

17.4 Didactic Workshop: How to Use Cards in Therapy

- **Suggested time:** 15 to 30 minutes in session (or as a homework between sessions).
- **Clear instructions:** choose recipient, write without self-censorship, then reread and edit, decide whether to share.
- **Subsequent exploration:** reading in a low voice, marking meaningful phrases, reflecting or discussing (according to emotional security).

- **Security guidelines:** advise the customer not to send the letter without processing it first, avoid it working as an ultimatum, have emotional support available.

- **Creative variants:**

    - Letter to the "future self" (an addiction-free self).
    - Letter to the "me of the past" (before consumption).
    - Letters in the third person (writing to substance as being).
    - Circulating between members of a family group with consent.

Potential risks and how to manage them

- Danger of emotional escalation if the letter is very aggressive or confrontational.

- If shared without preparation, it can lead to guilt, resentment, or negative feedback.

- It does not replace the therapeutic space but complements it.

- It should be used with clinical criteria: in cases of active crisis, it can intensify emotions if it is not modulated.

Follow-up activities and follow-up

- Share selected fragments in sessions and reflect in groups (when the dynamics allow it).

- Review a letter after a certain months to assess the internal change.

- Invite the use of continuous journals together with letters (combine continuous narrative with specific letters).

-Use as a trigger for thematic sessions (family, guilt, forgiveness, life projects).

CHAPTER 18
Books, Documentaries, and Resources that can Help You

A practical and motivating guide to continue learning and growing in your recovery.

18.1 Why Keep Learning?

We want to tell you something clear: your recovery does not end when you stop using. On the contrary, a new stage begins there. Learning about yourself, about addiction, about your brain, about how other people have coped, can help you better understand what is happening to you and how to move forward.

This chapter gives you **real resources**: books, documentaries, websites, and podcasts that have been helpful to many people like you. You don't need to read them all, just choose the ones that appeal to you the most. Each one can give you ideas, hope, or just make you feel like you're not alone.

18.2 Recommended Books

These books are not boring or full of difficult words. They are stories, ideas and knowledge that connect with real experience:

- *How to Change Your Mind*, by Michael Pollan.

He talks about how psychedelic therapies are being rediscovered (as part of a serious process) to treat depression, anxiety, and addiction. It's deep, but very accessible.

- *Chasing the Scream*, by Johann Hari.

A book that combines history, real cases and criticism of the "war on drugs" system. It makes you think about how the addict is punished instead of accompanying him.

- *In the Realm of Hungry Ghosts*, by Gabor Maté.

One of the most humane books about addiction. The author is a medical doctor and has worked with people in very difficult situations. Explain the pain behind addiction with compassion.

- *Recovery: Freedom from Our Addictions*, by Russell Brand.

A strong and honest testimony from someone who has been there. It uses humor, but it also offers concrete steps of recovery.

- Articles on therapeutic writing:

Not everything is heavy reading. There are articles (which you can ask your therapist for or look up online) that explain how writing letters or journals can help you organize your mind and process emotions.

18.3 Documentaries and Films to Reflect on

Sometimes seeing a true story impacts more than a thousand theories. These documentaries show you paths of recovery, relapses, hard decisions and also hope.

Title	What Is It About?	How Can It Help You?
Heroin(e)	Women fighting the opioid crisis	You'll see courage, compassion, and community
Recovery Boys	Young people in community treatment	It shows you that relapse is not the end of the road
Understanding the Opioid Epidemic	How the opioid crisis began	To understand what happens beyond the individual
One Little Pill	Alcoholism and an alternative medicine	Open your mind to other possible methods
Hamilton's Pharmacopeia	History and chemistry of substances	Knowing what you consume gives you power
Addiction (PBS / NOVA)	The Science of the Addicted Brain	Ideal if you are interested in the neurological part

How to use them?

- You can watch them alone, with a friend, your group, or therapist.
- Ask yourself questions like: What touched me? What made me angry? What reminded me of me?
- If you are in a group, you can debate: Which part best represents what I have experienced?

18.4 Online Resources

The Internet is full of noise, but also of good tools if you know how to search:

1- **Trusted addiction sites:** Look for pages of universities, hospitals, or specialized centers (not anonymous forums without moderation).

2- **Databases** such as PubMed (for scientific articles if you are interested in reading further).

3- **Podcasts:** There are series that interview people in recovery, therapists, psychiatrists, and family members. You can listen to them while walking or cooking.

4-**TED videos** on trauma, emotions, motivation, addictions.

5- **Secure *online* communities** (with supervision) such as SMART

Recovery, Reddit r/recovery or private groups on Facebook, if you are good at sharing.

18.5 How Do You Know if a Resource Is Good?

Not everything you see on social media or YouTube is reliable. To find out if it's worth it, look at this:

- Who wrote or recorded it? Is it someone with experience, training or real experience?
- Is it recent or very old?
- Is it based on facts, studies, science... or just opinions?

- Does it make you feel curious, wanting to know more... or makes you feel guilty or bad about yourself?

- Is it respectful, inclusive, open?

- Does it provide ideas that you can apply to your process?

18.6 What Do I Do with This Info Now?

Here are some practical ideas for integrating what you read or see:

- Choose **one reading or documentary per week** and make a summary for yourself or your therapist.

- Form a **"book club"** in your group or with friends who are in recovery.

- Pick an idea that has resonated with you and **write a letter to your "future self"** with what you learned.

- After watching or reading something, answer these three questions:

    - What idea left me thinking?
    - Which part did I identify with?
    - How might I apply this in my life?

Recovering is not only about giving up a substance. It is to build a life with meaning, knowledge, and tools. This chapter does not tell you what to do, it shows you possible paths. You are free to explore, try, leave and return. Because the most important thing is that you continue to learn to live, not just survive (figure 55).

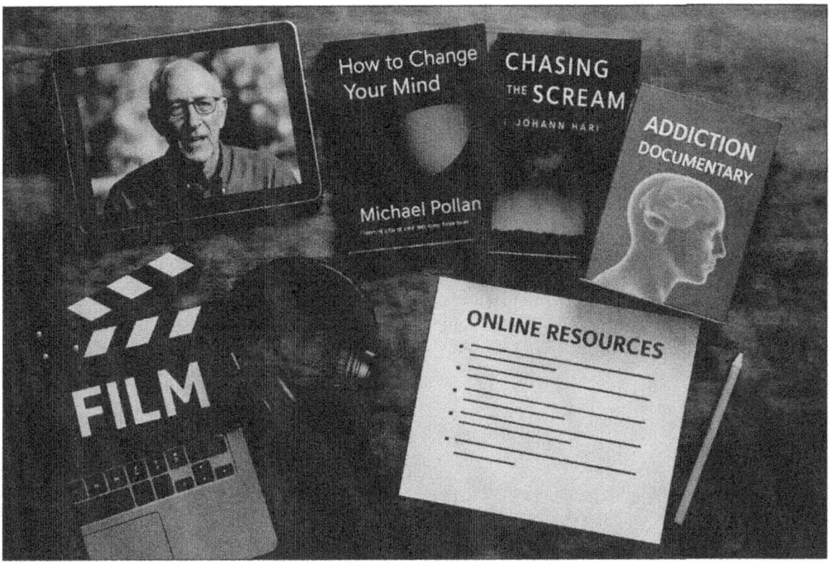

Figure 55. Movies, books, and online tools can help you understand your journey, feel accompanied, and discover new ways to move forward in your recovery. Exploring resources is also exploring your own transformation.

CHAPTER 19
The DNP-21 Model Applied to Addiction

19.1 What Is the DNP-21 Model?

The DNP-21 model (the predominant neurochemical domain of the 21$^{st.}$ century) arises in clinical practice, from the observation of hundreds of patients who did not respond to standard treatments. Based on these cases, recurrent patterns between symptoms and neurochemical profiles were identified, which allowed the design of an initial instrument capable of mapping dysfunctions in a systematic way.

This first instrument gave rise to U-DNP-21 (Universal DNP-21), a tool that generally evaluates all the neurochemical systems involved (DA, 5-HT, NE, GABA, Glutamate, ACh) and orients towards the predominant profile of each patient. Based on their results, the clinician can apply one of the six specific instruments of the model.

The DNP-21 model was conceived and developed by Dr. Alexis Gómez González, a clinical psychiatrist with training in neuroscience and advanced psychopharmacology (Cuba and Mexico). The proposal is nourished by years of medical practice, teaching and longitudinal follow-up of thousands of patients. The specialist combined scientific evidence with empathic observation and clinical criteria, as detailed on the www.dnp21.com website.

Together with Dr. Alexis Gómez González, the following have contributed to the development of the model:

- Clinical psychologists specialized in symptomatological evaluation.
- Neuropsychologists who collaborated in the design of cognitive sections of the instrument.
- Researchers in neuroimaging and pharmacodynamics.
- Volunteer patients, who contributed their experience, validation and experiential perspective.

19.2 Instrument AD-DNP-21-Addiction

Substance use disorders (SUD) and behavioral addictions (pathological gambling, compulsive use of networks, shopping, sex, among others) represent highly prevalent and complex clinical conditions. Beyond the moral or behavioral perspective, today they are understood as **neurobiological disorders** where the **dysregulation of multiple neurotransmitters** is central to their etiopathogenesis, course, and relapse.

The DNP-21 model allows for a personalized classification of the **predominant neurochemical profile** in patients with addiction, guiding therapeutic strategies based on individual neurochemical imbalance.

Neurobiological basis

Addictions not only acutely activate the reward system, but also produce chronic neuroadaptations that affect regions such as:

- Nucleus accumbens.
- Prefrontal cortex.
- Amygdala.
- Ventral tegmental area.
- Hippocampus.

These alterations mainly involve the following neurotransmitters:

Neurotransmitter	Impaired Function in Addiction
Dopamine (DA)	Reward Seeking, Motivation, Reinforcement
Glutamato (Glu)	Craving, dysfunctional associative learning
GABA	Anxiety, regulation of inhibitory control
Norepinephrine (NE)	Stress response, hypervigilance
Serotonina (5-HT)	Emotional regulation, impulsivity
Acetylcholine (ACh)	Reward Memory Encoding

Clinical Tool: AD-DNP-21 Questionnaire

The **AD-DNP-21 instrument** consists of **21 items distributed in six** neurochemical domains. Each item assesses relevant symptoms linked to specific neurotransmitters, on a scale of 0 to 3 points.

At the end, the most altered systems are identified and a personalized therapeutic plan is formulated.

Interpretation of the AD-DNP-21 Profile

The system with the highest score represents the predominant neurotransmitter (DNP) in that patient:

- DA-DNP-21 → Pathological motivation, maladaptive reinforcement.

- Glu-DNP-21 → Severe craving, lack of cognitive control.

- GABA-DNP-21 → Withdrawal anxiety, dysphoria.

- NE-DNP-21 → Hypervigilance, relapses in the context of stress.
- 5-HT-DNP-21 → Dysphoria, emotional impulsivity.
- ACh-DNP-21 → Intrusive memories, conditioned habits.

19.3 Clinical Cases

Case 1: DA-DNP-21–Cocaine

- A 32-year-old male. High impulsivity, anhedonia when discontinuing use, active search for gratification.
- Score: A 14, Glu 11, NE 8.
- Treatment: Bupropion + Intensive Motivational Therapy.

Case 2: GABA-DNP-21–Alcoholism

- A 45-year-old woman. Intense anticipatory anxiety, insomnia, physical dependence.
- Score: GABA 12, 5-HT 9, DA 7.
- Treatment: Gabapentin + CBT + mindfulness.

Case 3: ACh-DNP-21–Pathological Gambling

- A 29-year-old man. Intrusive thoughts, association of routines with play impulse.
- Score: ACh 11, DA 10, Glu 9.
- Treatment: Exposure therapy + Memantine (experimental).

Clinical Application and Projection

AD-DNP-21 makes it possible to segment clinical subtypes within the addictive spectrum, optimize pharmacological treatments and anticipate relapses according to the dominant system. Its systematic application offers a new standard in precision psychiatry for addiction.

19.4 AD-DNP-21-Neurochemical Profile Questionnaire in Addiction

Instructions:

Read each statement and mark with an X the option that best describes how often you have experienced this situation recently.

Scale:

0 = Never.

1 = Sometimes.

2 = Frequently.

3 = Almost always.

Affirmation	Never	Sometimes	Frequently	Almost always
1. I feel a strong need to seek immediate gratification.	☐	☐	☐	☐
2. Sometimes I consume or act just to feel "pleasure" or "euphoria".	☐	☐	☐	☐
3. I find it difficult to control pleasurable impulses even if it has negative consequences.	☐	☐	☐	☐
4. I feel like I need more to feel the same.	☐	☐	☐	☐
5. I become irritable if I Don't get what I want.	☐	☐	☐	☐
6. I have repetitive thoughts about consuming or repeating a behavior.	☐	☐	☐	☐
7. I feel impulsive and act without thinking.	☐	☐	☐	☐
8. When I try to let go of something, my mind won't leave me alone.	☐	☐	☐	☐
9. I feel intense anxiety when avoiding certain behaviors or substances.	☐	☐	☐	☐
10. I find it difficult to relax without resorting to a certain substance or behavior.	☐	☐	☐	☐
11. I get upset easily and then regret it.	☐	☐	☐	☐
12. I find it difficult to sleep or rest without outside help.	☐	☐	☐	☐
13. I feel in a constant state of alert.	☐	☐	☐	☐
14. I react with aggressiveness or irritability.	☐	☐	☐	☐
15. Under pressure or stress, I tend to relapse.	☐	☐	☐	☐
16. I feel sad or empty when I don't use or act as usual.	☐	☐	☐	☐
17. I feel guilty, shame, or hopelessness.	☐	☐	☐	☐

18. I use certain behaviors or substances to regulate my mood.	☐	☐	☐	☐
19. Everything reminds me of the addictive substance or behavior.	☐	☐	☐	☐
20. I have flashbacks, dreams, or intrusive thoughts.	☐	☐	☐	☐
21. I feel that certain routines or places trigger intense desires in me.	☐	☐	☐	☐

Key to Interpretation:

- Dopamine (DA) – Items 1–5: ________ (max. 15)
- Glutamato (Glu) – Ítems 6–9: ________ (máx. 12)
- GABA – Items 10–12: ________ (max. 9)
- Noradrenaline (NE) – Items 13–15: ________ (max. 9)
- Serotonin (5-HT) – Items 16–18: ________ (max. 9)
- Acetylcholine (ACh) – Items 19–21: ________ (max. 9)

DominantNeurochemicalProfile: ________________________

____

Suggested therapeutic recommendations: ____________

____

ProfessionalName: ________________________

____

Date: ________________________

Signature: ________________________

APPENDICES

Appendix 1
100 Frequently Asked Questions in My Consultation

Throughout my years of experience as a psychiatrist, I have accompanied people who struggle with different forms of addiction: substances, alcohol, compulsive behaviors, and even invisible forms of emotional dependence. I have also heard the suffering of their families, the bewilderment of their partners, and the frustration of health professionals seeking to understand and help.

This clinical practice has taught me that **addiction is not only a problem of consumption**, but a profound crisis of meaning, of the body, of emotional history and of the ability to bond with oneself and with others. It implies pain, but also a possibility of transformation.

This section brings together **the 100 most frequently asked questions that my patients, family and colleagues have asked me about addiction**. To make it easier for the reader to understand, I have organized the questions into thematic sections and answered them with clarity, scientific evidence, real examples and, above all, with compassion.

My purpose is not only to inform, but t**o offer a compass to those who feel lost** in the midst of this storm, showing that there are possible paths, tools and hopes.

I BASICS OF ADDICTION

1. What exactly is an addiction?

An addiction is a chronic disease of the brain that affects motivation, self-control, memory, and the reward system. It is not just a matter of consuming a substance or having a repetitive behavior, but of progressively losing the ability to decide. The person cannot stop doing so despite the physical, emotional, social or legal damage it causes.

2. When does consumption become an addiction?

When it stops being voluntary and begins to interfere with daily life. That is, when the desire or need to consume is stronger than the rational will. Also when there is tolerance (I need more to feel the same) or withdrawal syndrome (physical or emotional discomfort when leaving it).

3. Is dependence the same as addiction?

Not always. Physical dependence can occur with some medications (such as certain painkillers), without there being a compulsive desire to use them. Addiction involves compulsion, loss of control, and significant harm. But in practice, the two terms often go hand in hand.

4. Is addiction a choice or a disease?

It is not a simple choice. It's a complex disease that can start with a decision, but then hijacks brain circuits. No one chooses to have an addiction, just as no one chooses to have diabetes or depression. It requires treatment, not judgment.

5. Are all drugs equally addictive?

No. Some have a higher addictive potential than others. For example, nicotine, fentanyl, methamphetamine, and crack are highly addictive. Others, such as cannabis, can lead to addiction in certain contexts and vulnerable people.

6. Can you have addiction without using drugs?

Yes. There are behavioral addictions, such as pathological gambling, addiction to sex, technology, work or food. The brain mechanism is very similar: a repetitive behavior that activates the reward system and escapes voluntary control.

7. Is there a cure for addiction?

It does not have a "cure" in the classic sense, but it does have an effective treatment. Many people manage to live in full recovery, resume their lives and heal bonds. The key is to understand that it is a process, with possible relapses, but with many tools available.

8. Why do some people become addicted and others don't?

Many factors have an influence: genetic, emotional, traumatic, social and environmental. Childhood, attachment type, drug availability, unregulated emotions, and certain mental illnesses increase the risk. Addiction is not weakness: it is biological and emotional vulnerability.

9. Can an addicted person continue working or studying?

Yes, many functional people maintain activities, even without their surroundings noticing. But the emotional, physical, or relational toll is high. It's like driving a car with a damaged engine: you can move forward for a while, but you will end up failing.

10. Can addiction be prevented?

Yes. With healthy bonds, good emotional education, protective environments, clear boundaries and a less stressful society. Also detecting early signs of suffering in children, adolescents or adults who tend to seek relief in extreme substances or behaviors.

II HOW DOES AN ADDICTION START AND WHY?

11. Why do some people get hooked from the first time they consume?

Some substances immediately and powerfully activate the brain's reward system, releasing large amounts of dopamine. In people with genetic, emotional or psychological vulnerability, this "first click" can be so pleasurable or anesthetizing that they want to repeat it compulsively.

12. Do all addictions start with pleasure?

Not always. Many times they begin with avoidance, emotional pain or trauma. Some people use not to feel good, but to stop feeling bad. In those cases, the addiction is not born of pleasure, but of relief.

13. Can childhood trauma predispose to addiction?

Yes. Experiences of abuse, neglect, neglect, or unstable environments during childhood alter brain development, emotional regulation, and pain perception. Many addictions are unconscious attempts to soothe unhealed wounds.

14. Can a person become addicted without having traumatic factors?

Yes, although it is less frequent. Social environment, peer pressure, easy access to drugs, certain personality traits (impulsivity, anxiety), and unlimited recreational use can also lead to addiction.

15. What role does genetics play in addiction?

Genetics do not determine, but they predispose. Some people are born with increased sensitivity in their dopaminergic receptors or with lower tolerance to stress. If combined with negative environmental factors, the risk increases significantly.

16. Can occasional use lead to addiction?

Yes. What starts as something social or sporadic can become a necessity. The line between recreational use and addiction is thin, and many times it is crossed without the person realizing it.

17. What happens in the brain when an addiction is formed?

A hijacking of the reward circuit occurs. The brain begins to associate consumption with pleasure, relief or survival. Over time, other sources of satisfaction (family, achievements, relationships) lose emotional weight.

18. Why does someone continue to use if they know it hurts them?

Because addiction annuls the will. The conscious desire to stop is not enough when the body and brain are adapted to consumption. The person suffers from it, but cannot stop without help.

19. Does loneliness influence the development of an addiction?

A lot. Emotional loneliness, social disconnection or existential emptiness are frequent triggers. Addiction, in many cases, tries to fill a void or soothe an absence.

20. Is it true that we all have a potential addiction?

In a sense, yes. We are all looking to relieve pain, escape stress, or find pleasure. But not all of us have the same vulnerability. Recognizing our escape mechanisms is key to prevention.

III WARNING SIGNS IN ONESELF OR A LOVED ONE

21. How do I know if I have an addiction and not just a habit or custom?

The key difference is the loss of control. If you do it even if it hurts you, even if you want to stop and can't, even if it is affecting your personal, work or emotional life, it is no longer just a habit: it is an addiction.

22. What are the early signs that someone is developing an addiction?

- More frequent consumption or in greater quantities.
- Hiding or minimizing consumption.
- Unexplained mood swings.
- Isolation or irritability.
- Decline in work or academic performance.
- Denial and defensiveness when talking about the subject.

23. Is it normal for the person to deny that they have a problem

Yes. Denial is a common defense mechanism in addictions. It is not always a deliberate lie. Many times the person does not really realize the damage they are causing or is convinced that "they can leave whenever they want".

24. What do I do if I suspect a loved one has an addiction?

Observe without judgment, document worrisome behaviors, and approach from a place of care, not criticism. Express your concern with love, without accusing. Sometimes it's best to seek professional help before confronting directly.

25. Does addiction change a person's personality?

Yes, and sometimes in a very painful way. Addiction can make someone more aggressive, a liar, distant, or emotionally unstable. It is not because that person "no longer loves you", but because the substance alters their judgment, their affectivity and their priorities.

26. Can a functional person be living a covert addiction?

Yes. Many people keep their jobs, relationships, and routines, but secretly rely on a substance or behavior. It's known as "functional addiction," and it can last for years before the damage becomes apparent.

27. What behaviors indicate a possible relapse in someone who was already sober

- Irritability, isolation or insomnia.
- Neglect of routines or self-care.
- Avoid support groups or therapy.
- Small or evasive lies.
- Search for risky situations ("just one drink").

28. Can you help someone who doesn't want help?

It is very difficult, but not impossible. The first thing is not to give up or fall into despair. Sometimes change comes after a crisis or a loss. The most important thing is to stay present, set healthy boundaries and offer help without imposing it.

29. When should I consider a professional intervention?

When consumption severely affects health, safety, relationships, or daily functioning. Also if there have already been failed attempts to leave it or if there is a risk of harm to third parties. A well-guided intervention can save lives.

30. Can a person recover without admitting that they have a problem?

Not quite. Recognition is the first real step towards recovery. Without that awareness, it is difficult to sustain change. Some start treatment due to external pressure, but the best results occur when there is internal acceptance.

IV SPECIFIC SUBSTANCES AND THEIR EFFECTS

31. What is the most addictive drug out there?

It depends on the criteria (rapid addiction, harm, withdrawal). But among the most addictive are **nicotine**, **heroin/fentanyl**, **methamphetamine** and **alcohol**, due to their strong effect on the reward system and the withdrawal symptoms they generate.

32. Is it true that alcohol is more dangerous than some illegal drugs?

Yes. Although it is legal and socially accepted, alcohol is among the most harmful substances on a physical, emotional, and social level. It causes more deaths globally than many illegal drugs combined.

33. Can marijuana really be addictive?

Yes. Although many people consider it "natural" or "harmless", marijuana can lead to dependence, especially when consumed in excess, in adolescence, or with previous mental vulnerabilities.

34. What effects does cocaine have on the brain and body?

Cocaine produces intense euphoria, but short. It increases dopamine explosively. Its prolonged use damages the heart, the brain and can generate psychosis, paranoia or extreme anxiety.

35. Why is fentanyl so dangerous?

Because it is between 50 and 100 times more potent than morphine. Minimal doses are enough to cause overdose and death. In addition, it is mixed into drugs without the user knowing. It is a silent epidemic.

36. What are benzodiazepines and why do they cause addiction?

They are tranquilizers used for anxiety or insomnia (e.g., alprazolam, clonazepam). They can generate **physical and psychological dependence** if used for a long time or without medical supervision. Withdrawal can be severe.

37. What about methamphetamines? Why are they so destructive?

Methamphetamines overactivate the alert and pleasure system. They cause euphoria, insomnia, aggressiveness and accelerated physical deterioration. In the long term, they can damage the brain irreversibly.

38. What effects does drug use have on mental health?

Drugs can **trigger or worsen mental disorders**, such as depression, anxiety, psychosis, or bipolar disorder. They also generate an emotional roller coaster, which makes diagnosis and treatment difficult.

39. What happens when several drugs are combined (polyconsumption)?

Polydrug use enhances risks. Some combinations (alcohol + benzodiazepines, opioids + stimulants) can be deadly. The body is not prepared to handle so many contradictory effects at once.

40. What do I do if I suspect a family member is using drugs, but they don't tell me?

Avoid aggressive confrontations. Observe carefully, look for calm moments to talk, and express your concern from love, not fear or accusation. Sometimes it's best to see an addiction specialist to guide the conversation.

V NON-SUBSTANCE ADDICTIONS (TECHNOLOGY, FOOD, SEX AND GAMBLING)

41. What is a non-substance addiction?

It is a repetitive and compulsive behavior that, without involving a chemical substance, activates the brain's reward system and generates loss of control. Common examples: pathological gambling, compulsive shopping, excessive use of social networks, food, sex.

42. Is cell phone or social media addiction real?

Yes. Constant interaction with notifications, likes, and visual stimuli activates dopamine, reinforces the need for connection, and can interfere with concentration, sleep, and emotional health.

43. Can emotional eating be a form of addiction?

Yes. Many people use food as an emotional anesthetic. "Binge eating" or compulsion for certain foods is often related to anxiety, trauma, or low self-esteem.

44. How do I know if I have an addiction to sex or pornography?

If the urge is uncontrollable, interferes with your daily life, causes guilt or isolation, or you need higher and higher levels of stimulation to feel the same, an addictive pattern may be present.

45. Why does gambling (gambling, casinos, aps) generate so much addiction?

Because it combines chance, the promise of immediate reward and the activation of dopamine. Losses also reinforce the cycle ("next time I get back what I lost"). It is a very powerful psychological and neurochemical trap.

46. Can compulsive shopping be considered an addiction?

Yes. Many people buy to calm emotions, fill gaps or avoid problems. The feeling of relief is temporary and often followed by guilt or financial problems.

47. Why are these addictions more invisible or less understood?

Because they do not involve illegal substances, they are socially normalized or even valued (such as working hard, being connected, being "fit"). But they can cause the same level of suffering and deterioration.

48. Are they treated the same as substance addictions?

In many respects yes: psychotherapy, emotional regulation, change of habits and social support are required. Sometimes there are complementary pharmacological treatments if they coexist with depression or anxiety.

49. What role does shame play in these addictions?

A central role. Many people feel "weak", "ridiculous", or "sick" because they can't control their behavior. Shame fuels isolation and makes it difficult to ask for help.

50. Can a non-substance addiction be as serious as a drug addiction?

Yes. Even if there is no physical overdose, the emotional, relational, work or psychological damage can be equal or even greater. All addiction is suffering that deserves attention and treatment.

VI NEUROBIOLOGY OF THE ADDICTED BRAIN

51. What happens in the brain when an addiction develops?

The reward system is altered, especially the dopaminergic pathway. The substance or behavior is associated with pleasure or relief, and the brain begins to prioritize it over other needs. There is a hijacking of voluntary control.

52. What is dopamine and why is it so important in addiction?

It is a neurotransmitter that regulates pleasure, motivation, and learning. In addiction, dopamine levels are artificially triggered. The brain adapts and stops responding to natural stimuli (food, affection, achievements).

53. Why do you lose control if the brain "knows" that it is doing harm?

Because the rational system (prefrontal cortex) is weakened, while the reward system and the impulse (limbic system) dominate. Knowing does not always imply being able to act.

54. Does addiction leave permanent brain damage?

It depends on the type of substance, the duration of consumption, and the age of onset. Some drugs such as alcohol, methamphetamines, or inhalants can cause structural damage. But many functions can improve with time and abstinence.

55. Why do some people relapse even after years of soberness?

Because the brain retains "traces" of addiction. Certain contexts, emotions or stimuli can reactivate these memories. Relapse is not always a lack of will, but part of the neuroadaptive process.

56. What is tolerance?

It is the need to consume larger amounts to obtain the same effect. The brain adapts to the repeated stimulus, and no longer responds in the same way. Tolerance is a key signal of neuroadaptation.

57. What about the withdrawal syndrome?

It is the set of physical and emotional symptoms that appear when the substance is stopped. They can include tremors, anxiety, insomnia, depression, physical pain, or seizures, depending on the type of drug.

58. Is a teenager's brain more vulnerable to addiction?

Yes. The adolescent brain is still developing, especially the prefrontal cortex (control, judgment). This makes them more impulsive and less aware of risk, which increases the likelihood of addiction.

59. What other neurotransmitters are involved in addiction?

In addition to dopamine, serotonin (mood), GABA (inhibition), glutamate (learning), and endorphins (natural pleasure) are involved. All of these systems are altered during an addiction.

60. Can the addicted brain recover?

Yes. Although some scars remain, the brain has plasticity: the ability to regenerate connections, change habits, and learn new forms of self-regulation. Treatment and timing make a real difference.

VII MEDICAL AND PHARMACOLOGICAL TREATMENTS

61. Are there medications that help you quit drugs?

Yes. Some medications can reduce craving, relieve withdrawal, or block the pleasurable effects of certain substances. They do not cure addiction, but they facilitate the recovery process.

62. What medications are used to quit alcohol?

They can be used:

- Naltrexone: reduces the desire to drink.
- Acamprosate: helps maintain abstinence.

- Disulfiram: causes unpleasant effects if drunk.

-Temporary anxiolytics and vitamins (such as thiamine) in detoxification.

63. What about addiction to opioids such as heroin or fentanyl?

- Methadone and buprenorphine: replace the opioid in a controlled manner.

- Naltrexone: blocks the effects of the drug.

- Clonidine: helps with withdrawal symptoms.

These treatments must be done under specialized medical supervision.

64. Are there medications to quit smoking?

Yes. The most commonly used are:

-Bupropion: antidepressant that reduces anxiety and desire.

-Varenicline: acts on nicotinic receptors.

- Nicotine patches, gum, or sprays as replacement therapy.

65. Are there medications for cocaine addiction or methamphetamines?

There are currently no specific drugs approved for these substances, but some antidepressants, mood stabilizers, and ADHD medications may help in certain cases. **The psychological approach is key**.

66. Do these medications cause addiction?

Most do not. Some may have the potential for abuse if misused, such as benzodiazepines. That is why they should be used only under medical indication and follow-up, as part of a comprehensive treatment plan.

67. Is it necessary to be hospitalized to receive medical treatment?

Not always. It depends on the degree of addiction, medical risks, family environment and motivation of the patient. There are **outpatient options, day clinics and short hospitalizations** depending on the case.

68. Is medical treatment sufficient on its own?

No. It is a **part of the comprehensive treatment**. Without psychological support, life changes and emotional containment, medications may not be enough. Addiction is biopsychosocial, and should be treated as such.

69. What happens if a patient refuses to take medication?

It is important **to respect their decision** and explore other forms of help. Sometimes rejection is due to fear, bad experiences, or stigma. Therapeutic alliance and education can open new doors.

70. How long should pharmacological treatment last?

It varies according to each case. Some medications are used only in detoxification, others for months or years. Ideally, it should be **evaluated periodically with the clinical team** and adapted to the patient's evolution.

VIII PSYCHOLOGICAL THERAPIES AND EMOTIONAL APPROACH

71. Does psychotherapy really help in addiction?

Yes. It is one of the pillars of treatment. Therapy not only works on addictive behavior, but also on the emotions, traumas, beliefs, bonds and meaning of life that are behind consumption.

72. What type of therapy is the most recommended?

The most effective include:

-Cognitive behavioral therapy (CBT).

-Dialectical-behavioral therapy (DBT).

-EMDR (for trauma).

-Mindfulness and third-generation therapies.

The choice depends on the patient's profile.

73. Is group therapy helpful?

Yes. It helps break isolation, normalize suffering, and build a support network. Listening to others allows you to see your own problem more clearly and feel accompanied.

74. How do you work on relapses in therapy?

Without punishment or guilt. The factors **that led to relapse are analyzed, early signs are identified, and tools to prevent further falls are reinforced. Every relapse is also a lesson**.

75. Is it necessary to talk about the past and childhood?

Many times yes. Addiction is often a symptom of unhealed wounds. Understanding the emotional history helps to stop repeating patterns and to build new forms of self-regulation.

76. What do I do if I have a hard time trusting therapists?

It's normal. Many people have been hurt or judged. The therapeutic relationship is built step by step, without pressure. Looking for a professional with whom you have a connection is key.

77. How do you work on the emotional void left by addiction?

New sources of pleasure, meaning and connection are built. Recovery is not just about leaving something, but filling that space with something authentic and restorative: bonds, projects, spirituality, art, purpose.

78. Does therapy work even if the person does not want to quit the addiction?

It can be helpful. Sometimes the process begins with ambivalent exploration: "one part of me wants, another part doesn't." Validating that internal conflict can open the door to genuine change.

79. How long should psychological treatment be?

There is no fixed duration. Some people need a few months; others, years. The important thing is that the process is deep, flexible and adapted to the patient's rhythm.

80. What happens if I start to feel worse at the beginning of therapy?

It's common. By removing layers of denial, intense emotions can arise. It is a sign that the inner work is beginning. It is not a step backwards, but part of the healing process.

IX REHABILITATION, RELAPSE, AND RECOVERY

81. What does it really mean to "be in recovery"?

It is not only about stopping using, but about transforming one's relationship with oneself, with pain, with pleasure and with life. To recover is to learn to live without escaping, without numbing, without destroying.

82. Is recovery possible for everyone?

Yes. Although the road is difficult, every person has the capacity for change, resilience and reconstruction. Even those who have relapsed many times can get back up and find a new life.

83. What is a therapeutic community or rehabilitation center?

It is a residential space where the person receives intensive treatment. It combines psychotherapy, workshops, daily structure, group activities and professional accompaniment. It's not confinement, it's containment.

84. Do all people need hospitalization?

No. Treatment should be appropriate to the level of risk, family support and motivation. Many people can recover with outpatient care. Internment is not punishment: it is just another therapeutic tool.

85. How is a relapse managed?

With understanding and strategy. It is not a matter of "starting from scratch", but of reviewing what went wrong, adjusting the treatment and moving forward. Relapses are part of the process, not the end of it.

86. Why are relapses so frequent?

Because addiction leaves deep traces. Stress, sadness, isolation or contact with the previous environment can activate desire. Recovering also implies preventing and managing these moments of vulnerability.

87. What is a support network and why is it so important?

It is the set of people and resources that support the patient emotionally: family, friends, groups, therapists. A solid support network protects against relapse and accompanies you in difficult times.

88. Can one live fully without ever consuming again?

Yes. Many people achieve a sober, creative, loving, and free life. The key is not only to abstain, but to build a life project with meaning, connection and authentic satisfaction.

89. How to maintain motivation over time?

Celebrating achievements, connecting with personal values, participating in groups, helping others. Motivation is not constant, but it can be renewed when it is transformed into purpose.

90. Does recovery have an end or is it forever?

Recovery is an ongoing process, not a static goal. It does not mean to be "healed", but to be on a journey, attentive, present, free. Some say: "it's not a finish line, it's a way of life".

X IMPACT ON THE FAMILY, STIGMA AND PATHS OF HOPE

91. How does addiction affect the family?

Deeply. It generates pain, confusion, anger, guilt, fear and ruptures. The family often becomes a caregiver, victim and silent witness to deterioration. It can also be an active part of recovery.

92. What is codependency?

It is a dynamic in which the family member annuls himself to "sabe" the addict. He lives aware of his behavior, blames himself for his relapse or covers it up. Breaking this dynamic is critical to healing both.

93. What can I do if my loved one does not accept help?

Set firm and loving limits, take care of your well-being, and do not feed denial. Sometimes the person hits rock bottom before asking for help. In the meantime, you can also seek support for yourself.

94. Should I forgive someone who has lied or hurt because of their addiction?

Forgiveness is a personal process. It does not mean justifying, but freeing yourself from resentment. You can set boundaries and take care of your dignity, but also open space for compassion if you wish.

95. Does society judge those who have an addiction too much?

Yes, there is a lot of stigma, discrimination and ignorance. It is believed to be a "vice" or a "decisión", when in fact it is a complex disease. Humanizing addiction is an urgent social task.

96. Can spirituality help in recovery?

Yes. It's not necessarily about religion, but about reconnecting with something bigger than pain: meaning, purpose, transcendence, inner connection. Spirituality can be a profound pillar of change.

97. What is a "day at a time"?

It is a fundamental principle in recovery: not to anticipate the entire future, but to focus on the present. Every sober day is a victory. Each conscious moment is one more step.

98. Can I help others if I too have gone through an addiction?

Yes! Many of the best guides are people in recovery. Her testimony has strength, empathy and truth. Helping others also strengthens your own path.

99. What can I do if I relapse and feel defeated?

Don't beat yourself up. Falling doesn't erase what you've advanced. Ask for help, talk, start again. Every relapse is an opportunity to come back more aware, wiser, and stronger.

100. Is it worth fighting to get out of addiction?

Yes, always. Although it may seem impossible, there is life beyond consumption, beyond pain, beyond the past. Recovery isn't just possible: it can be the beginning of something you never thought you had.

Illustrated Glossary of Terms on Addiction

Language shapes the way we understand addiction. Many technical, clinical, or popular terms can be confusing, stigmatizing, or misused. This illustrated glossary seeks to clarify the most important concepts related to the world of addictions, explained in a simple way and accompanied by symbolic images that help to understand and reflect on them.

Why an illustrated glossary?

- **Accessible comprehension:** Not all readers have medical or psychological training. The goal is to translate complex terms into clear, visual language.
- **Combating stigma:** Explaining terms avoids negative labels such as "vicious", "weak" or "hopelessly ill".
- **Visual memory:** Illustrations allow you to better remember concepts and connect them emotionally.

Key Terms (Examples)

Addiction

Definition: Chronic disease characterized by the compulsive pursuit of a substance or behavior, despite its negative consequences.

Symbolic illustration: A figure trapped in a labyrinth that he feeds himself, but seeks a way out.

Tolerance

Definition: The need to increase the dose of a substance to obtain the same effect.

Symbolic illustration: A staircase that extends upwards while the effect remains at the base.

Withdrawal syndrome

Definition: A set of physical and emotional symptoms that appear when a substance is abruptly reduced or stopped.
Symbolic illustration: A body in shadow, trembling as a wave violently recedes.

Relapse

Definition: Return to consumption after a period of abstinence. It is not a failure, but a common part of the recovery process.
Symbolic illustration: A walker who stumbles on the path, but gets up with help.

Codependency

Definition: Dysfunctional relationship pattern where one person revolves his or her life around another's problem.
Symbolic illustration: Two figures joined by a rope, one dragging the other.

Support Network

Definition: Group of people, resources, or institutions that provide emotional and practical support to those seeking recovery.
Symbolic illustration: Several hands holding a single hand, which ascends towards the light.

Harm Reduction

Definition: Public health strategy that seeks to reduce the negative effects of consumption, without requiring abstinence as the only objective.

Symbolic illustration: A parachute deployed, smoothing out a fall.

Double diagnosis

Definition: Simultaneous presence of a substance use disorder and another mental disorder (such as depression, anxiety, bipolar disorder, etc.).

Symbolic illustration: A broken mirror with two superimposed reflections.

Psychoactive substances

Definition: Substances that affect the central nervous system and modify mood, perception, or behavior.

Examples: Alcohol, cannabis, cocaine, benzodiazepines, tobacco, caffeine.

Symbolic illustration: A brain surrounded by small bubbles with icons of each substance.

Neuroadaptation

Definition: Progressive changes in the brain as a result of repeated use, which modify brain chemistry and reinforce addiction.

Symbolic illustration: A neural circuit that becomes entangled like a spider's web.

Recommendations for using this glossary

- Ideal for educational sessions with patients, family members or students.
- It can be used as a visual aid in workshops, therapies or conferences.
- Useful as preventive material in schools and communities.
- Designed to encourage dialogue and demystify addiction.

Telegalenos a gabacha quitá Collection

A Compassionate, Scientific, and Practical Guide to Facing the Challenges of the Mind and Soul.

The collection *Telegalenos a gabacha quitá* was born with a clear mission: **to accompany, inform and alleviate**. Each volume is dedicated to a specific mental health condition, and becomes an intimate conversation between the reader and the psychiatrist. With accessible yet rigorously scientific language, the books address symptoms, causes, treatments, myths, and possibilities for recovery.

More than just manuals, these texts integrate the perspective of medical aikido, a humanistic and dynamic approach to transforming emotional suffering into inner strength. In addition, each book includes up-to-date directories of **sources of help in Mexico, Spain, and the United States**, and offers real bridges to treatment and community accompaniment.

If you found this book about **addiction useful or revealing, we invite you to discover the other titles in the collection**:

Depression

"The body is silent about what the soul cannot express". This book explores the neurochemical mechanisms, emotional wounds, and social circumstances that can lead to a depressive state. Its pages offer everything from diagnostic criteria to integrative interventions: pharmacological, psychotherapeutic, somatic and spiritual. It includes emotional regulation techniques, help resources in three countries and a special chapter on how to accompany those who suffer without falling into judgment or despair.

Anxiety

"When the alarm system never goes off". This book walks you through the different forms of anxiety—generalized, panic, phobic, social—and their effects on the body and mind. It offers practical tools such as somatic breathing, graded exposures, mindfulness, and pharmacotherapy. With a medical aikido approach, you will learn how to transform anxiety into channeled life energy and seek timely help when fear becomes chronic.

ADHD

"It's not a lack of will, it's a brain that works differently". An essential book for parents, diagnosed adults and professionals. It presents current scientific studies, pharmacological options (such as methylphenidate and atomoxetine), school accommodations, and behavioral therapies. In addition, it explores how to channel the energy of ADHD into creativity, compassionate organization, and self-understanding through mental aikido techniques.

Dementia

"Memory fades, but love remains". A warm and scientific guide for those living with dementia and their caregivers. The book addresses Alzheimer's, frontotemporal dementia, vascular dementia and Lewy bodies with diagnostic criteria, non-pharmacological strategies, legal guidance, behavior management and emotional containment of the caregiver. Medical aikido proposes a way to accompany with respect, dignity and deep connection.

Insomnia

"Sleeping is not giving up, it is an act of Health". Chronic insomnia is a silent epidemic. Here you'll discover the neurobiological causes, dysfunctional beliefs that perpetuate it, and the most effective strategies for catching up on sleep, such as cognitive behavioral therapy for insomnia (CBT-I), sleep hygiene, body relaxation techniques, and pharmacological alternatives when needed.

Schizophrenia

"Seeing another reality is not madness, it is suffering on another frequency". Clinically sensitive and non-sensational, this book explains the positive and negative symptoms, the evolution of the disorder, current drug treatments, psychosocial approaches, and how support networks can make a difference. Through medical aikido, schizophrenia is approached as a struggle for internal coherence, where it is possible to accompany without fear and with meaning.

Bipolarity

"Between euphoria and hopelessness, there is also balance". It clearly describes manic, depressive, and mixed episodes, treatments with mood stabilizers (such as lithium, valproate, and lamotrigine), the most common triggers, and the changes needed to sustain a functional life. It includes guidelines for family members, relapse prevention, and mind-body integrative strategies to regain center in the midst of emotional chaos.

Autism

This book is not about "correcting" an autistic child... try to understand it. Every autistic mind deserves a world that understands it. It is a warm, clear, and hope-filled guide for families seeking real answers, professionals who want to learn, and autistic adults who deserve to be heard. It's a journey into the most beautiful thing about neurodevelopment: authenticity. It is not a manual. It is not a diagnosis. It's a hug.

Why choose this collection?

- Because it is written by a clinical psychiatrist with experience in consultation, emergencies and therapy.
- Because it is based on up-to-date scientific studies and international guidelines.
- Because it has an understandable language, without losing scientific precision.
- Because it includes non-pharmacological approaches, integrative medicine, and spirituality.
- Because it integrates the model of medical aikido: anticipate, contain, transform.
- Because it provides real help resources in three countries: Mexico, Spain, and the United States.
- Because it was designed for patients, family members and professionals.

Explore, understand and accompany. *Telegalenos a gabacha quitá* is more than a collection of books: it is a community of knowledge, compassion, and possibility.